Red Earth Wisdom

Red Earth Wisdom

on healing your life

BY LINDA S. BOWLBY, M.D.

PSYCHIATRIST

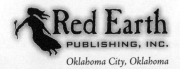

Red Earth

PUBLISHING, INC.

Oklahoma City, Oklahoma

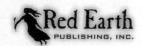

Copyright 2006 by Red Earth Publishing, Inc./www.redearthwisdom.com

Printed in the United States of America.
ISBN 0-9779993-0-0
Library of Congress Catalog Number 2006927927
Cover and contents designed by Sandi Welch/www.2WDesignGroup.com
Cover photo of Antelope canyon, located in northcentral Arizona, by Linda Bowlby.

CONTENTS

Many names have been changed
to protect the anonymity of those concerned.

This manuscript is a compilation of essays written from 1996-2001, and Dr. Bowlby has kept the present tense in these writings to remain true to the spirit in which they were written.

INTRODUCTION

HAVING SURVIVED AND HEALED from childhood satanic abuse, I know to the depth of my being that no matter what your pain you can heal. In healing, I traveled to the center of my being, remembered my childhood trauma, and released the anger, fear, and pain that bound me. On my inward journey, I found God, the source of all power and wisdom.

My healing required daily prayer and meditation. In the silence, I learned to listen for and trust the Divine Voice that came in the form of an intuitive knowing or an inner voice that resonated truth. Centered in daily communion with God, my eyes and ears were open to see, hear, and learn from God's abundant messengers and teachers, who often came to me in the most earthy of costumes.

Rooted in Oklahoma's rich red earth, I am a woman that has traversed her pain into healing. In that pain, I found my true source of wisdom—God. I found God within me, within you, and throughout the planet.

In my healing, I learned that our minds are extraordinarily powerful and what we choose to think determines our feelings, actions, and health. I also learned that our life's purpose is to evolve spiritually and to help others to evolve spiritually. For our higher good and the higher good of the planet, we each must choose to align our thoughts and actions with the Universal Divine.

My message is a simple one. To find God, go within. Rely on God's strength to feel and release your emotional baggage. Choose positive, loving, life-affirming thoughts to heal your body, mind, and spirit. Then, help others.

PART ONE

Wisdom's Teachers

CHAPTER ONE

Born Country

In my youth, I was oblivious to the wisdom and teachers found in my rural Oklahoma home, because in the words of a Barbara Mandrell song, "I was country, when country wasn't cool." I grew up ashamed of my country heritage. I thought country humor and life were rude and crude, and I did my best to educate the country right out of me.

Too often, regardless of our heritage—be it Polish, Jewish, African, Asian, rural, urban, east, west, north, or south of the proverbial tracks—we feel embarrassed or ashamed of our birth origins. As part of our health and healing, we must embrace our heritage and come to know it gives us grounding and depth. If we reject our origins, we reject ourselves.

In my maturation and healing, I grew to appreciate and value the fact that country folks have common sense, down-to-earth ways, and a belly-laughing sense of the absurd. Being reared in the country, I did not value rural wisdom until I became "educated."

As a child and adolescent, I just knew when I got to the "big city" and college the wisdom of the world would open to me, and it did, but not in the way I expected. The city and college often taught by negative example. After those lessons, I came to value my country teachers.

We of the Western world exhaustively look to books, schools, and gurus for answers. We too often go around with our heads in the clouds and miss wisdom's teachers found in everyday life.

Barney is one of my rural teachers. One July, we Oklahomans were experiencing our twentieth-plus day of one-hundred-degree weather. I commented on the heat to Barney, the feed store owner. As he stood there in overalls, surrounded by bags of seed, feed, and fertilizer, this wizened old man with his big tobaccy smile said, "We got to take the bad with the good."

Each time I go to Barney for dog and chicken food, I come away with a smile. Barney just does that for people. He is always joking, giving you something, or telling you his most recent remedy. Barney uses a lot of horse liniment.

When my eyes and ears are open, my teachers abound. I used to have my hair cut in a rural barber shop. As the barber clipped my hair, I loved to listen to the farmers in the adjacent chairs talk of sports, crops, weather, and the local gossip. There was nothing fancy about these men. They were pure country. They spit, drove pick-up trucks, and wore overalls or cowboy shirts and blue-jeans.

Now, if you only listened to television and media hype, you would believe these people no longer existed but, if you drive across America, you will see them everywhere. These country folks are there in the wide open spaces, which also still exist.

They grow your food, run your factories, and keep America going. These people still believe in mom and apple pie, love and family, and church on Sunday.

No matter how much the media glorifies war, crime, sex, and computers, America's heartland still exists, and this heart of our land is occupied by wise teachers, like those good ol' boys I met occupying the next barber chair.

PRETENSIONS

People teach me so much with the words they choose to use and often amaze me in their pretentious words and trappings. A friend and I often laugh and call my farm—a collection of chicken and generator houses, barn, and home—a "country estate" and the "Bowlby Compound," and my collection of Heinz 57 dogs a "kennel." The words "estate, compound, and kennel" imply exclusivity and elitism, but the words "farm, dogs, and chicken house" speak of plain country living.

I see such pretentious trappings as I drive to and from the city and pass exclusive homes with grounds, computerized gates, and square footage requiring roller skates for navigation and an uncle in the electric company. I muse on the follies of the human ego.

Pretensions are based on feelings of fear and insecurity. Pretentious people have a fear of not being "good enough," whatever that is. Usually the "good enough" standard is established by a mythical set of rules, most often conveyed to us through advertising, television, and long forgotten messages. These standards are unattainable by most, if not all, humans. Those who feel secure in themselves have little need to impress anyone with their clothes, house, car, or neighborhood. Secure individuals have no need for a facade. They know who they are is more valuable than anyone they could pretend to be.

When we chase these mythical standards, the needs of our spirit go unattended. We are in disharmony with our essence. When we find ourselves using pretentious words like "estates, compounds, and kennels," we need to look within. What do we fear? Who are we trying to impress? Are we being true to ourselves? If the latter answer is no, then state the truth of whatever reality you are trying to glorify, even if it is a chicken house, barn, or Heinz 57 dogs. Join the human race. Get emotionally naked. Go skinny dipping.

I heard a similar message one day as I was speeding down the road, in my old brown truck, toward a rural Oklahoma clinic. I listened as Jann Browne belted out a tune, "You Ain't Down-Home."

She sings of individuals who know the "right people," wear the "right clothes," drive "snappy little sports cars," and have "cool conversations" on their "high-tech telephones." Then she belts out they've got "one little problem:" they "ain't down-home." They "ain't down-home where the people got their feet on the ground" and "where there is plenty of love to go 'round."

She goes on to sing that they have brand new Jacuzzis, gold credit cards, and are known in every "high-class place in town," but, again, she belts, they've got "one little problem," they "ain't down-home."

Jann's tune carries the wisdom of casting off the pretentious and irrelevant and embracing our true or divine Selves. Are you down home?

◎ ◎ ◎

In our world, teachers abound. They are not confined to the towers of education and learning. In fact, they are too infrequently found there. Most often our teachers are the people we meet in everyday life, the words they use, and the behaviors they exhibit.

Our teachers also come from our origins. within every culture there is deep fundamental wisdom and truth.

Yet our greatest teacher comes from within, that inner voice, our connection with the Divine. To that voice we must be true and, with that voice, all other information we incorporate into our being must resonate.

As for me, I now embrace my heritage and am grateful that "I was country, when country wasn't cool."

CHAPTER TWO

Pet Teachers

OVER THE YEARS, I'VE HAD AN ASSORTMENT OF PETS, and they have been my teachers. During one year on the farm, over twenty dogs found their way to me. These were above my own crew in residence. I tended each new arrival, and they eventually were adopted into my brood or taken to the local pet adoption center.

I have a neighbor who will shoot the strays if he finds them first. I do not understand his cruelty and that of those who abandon their animals, especially when there are kindly adoption centers where children and adults alike delight in receiving new pets.

I believe animals are of divine origins and connecting with them heals the soul.

MAMA

With man's proclivity for abandonment, when I think I hear squeals of puppies, I had better go look. "Mama" came to me that way.

It had stormed that night. Warmly tucked in bed, I heard

what I took to be coyotes, but I thought they were unusually close to the house. I later heard an unfamiliar dog bark.

The next morning, I again heard the strange bark. When I investigated, I discovered a mother and eight puppies. From the markings of five of the puppies, I thought the father was a rottweiler, but I puzzled over the lineage of the mother. She was ferocious in protecting her babies. I left her food that morning. The following morning, I left her more food.

As I was giving her and her babies a wide berth, the mother approached me and allowed me to pet her. As I stroked her broad tawny head, I called her "Mama." I told her what a good job she had done caring for her babies. I felt her exhaustion, and the look in her eyes thanked me for caring for her and her children. We were one mother to another. As the days passed, I watched Mama protect food and territory from my other dogs. She vigilantly herded her frolicking six-to-eight-week-old flock.

I was awed by Mama's incredibly muscular body and observed healed angular gashes about her neck. I felt overwhelmed in my desire to keep all of this family of nine.

Later, a friend informed me this ferocious muscular mother was a pit bull. I knew then it would be unsafe for all concerned to allow her and her babies to roam free on my farm.

I decided to keep Caroline, with rottweiler markings. I felt sad and cried when a friend took Mama and the other babies to find new homes. I have often grieved Mama and wished I had kept her because, for a brief moment in time, we communed in that universal bond of one mother to another.

BETH

After suffering abuse and neglect, Beth was abandoned and found her way to my farm. Beth is black, with white facial markings and wounded dark-brown eyes. She is of unknown birth origins and has been a most amazing teacher.

When I return home from work, my dogs greet me en masse. If one is missing, their absence alerts my concern and frequently means they are dead from either animal or human encounter. One winter, for two nights Beth had not greeted me with the other dogs. The morning after the second night, she slowly approached me limping, with a strange appearance to her neck. As I bent to pet and examine her, I was confronted by a grapefruit-sized gaping wound encompassing half of her neck. Her splayed flesh revealed her neck musculature and intact major blood vessels. At first, I recoiled and thought of the veterinarian. After gathering my wits, I remembered how Beth was terrorized by a routine visit to the veterinarian, and I knew she would be traumatized if I took her into town to see him.

Quickly, I reviewed my surgical skills gleaned from three dreadful months on the surgery service in medical school. I collected peroxide, alcohol, iodine, bandages, and hot water. I had seen wounds of that size heal from the base, without suturing.

As I softly talked and crooned to her, Beth lay on her side while I proceeded to cleanse her deep angry wound. Without anesthetic, only occasionally whimpering, she patiently allowed me to touch deep into her flesh and remove particles of grass and debris.

As I worked, I felt one with the countrywomen of old. When they tended their wounded animals, husbands, and children, they had no doctors or pharmacies. They reached deep into themselves and their ancient wisdom. I reflected how tending the sick and wounded had always been a woman's task, long before men began to call themselves "doctors."

After Beth was bandaged, I gave her a penicillin shot. She ate, took liquids, and rested in the house near the wood stove, where she lay quietly for two days. On the third day, I came home from work to find that Beth had torn screens from windows and doors in attempts to get outside. As hard as it was, I set her free.

In spite of my best efforts at bandaging, after a few days I gave up trying to keep her raw flesh covered. Daily, I tended her wound with peroxide and iodine. The other dogs, and with contorted efforts Beth herself, added their therapeutic touch by licking her raw wound. As unclean as it seems, nature's wisdom prevailed. The dogs' saliva contains antibodies.

While healing, Beth stayed to herself, lying in the tall grass away from the house and the other dogs. Beth wisely knew she needed fresh air, an open clean wound, rest, and occasional exercise.

I watched in awe as Beth's gaping wound slowly scarred and shrank to the size of a quarter and then closed itself, proving once more that God and Nature heal, man only tends.

I was deeply touched and have long marveled, after a fatal wound for most dogs, Beth had the fortitude to live and make her way home. I believe in a deep primal way our love for each other drew her back to me, where she knew she would be safe and tended.

WILLIE

Willie was a black woolly chow that appeared on my farm. He was skittish around people and had obviously been abused. Of course, right away, he pulled on my heartstrings, but goodness that dog was ugly. Since he was the new kid on the block, my other dogs bullied Willie. I talked to them and to Willie, attempting to settle down the crew. I gave Willie some time to see if he was a fit, but goodness, that dog was ugly. After Willie stayed several weeks, it was clear the other dogs would not accept him. For his well being, I found him a new home, but by the time he left, I had come to care for Willie, and he no longer seemed ugly. I had come to see Willie with my heart and not my eyes.

CHICKENS AND PUPPIES

One November when my son Jeffrey was twelve, he incubated, with the assistance of a heat lamp, a dozen chicken eggs in his bedroom. Two weeks later out came Fred and Mollie. While waiting for the expected hatchings, Jeffrey and I constructed a chicken house.

While Fred and Mollie were residing in my living room in the process of growing and going from fuzz to feathers, we discovered we had waited too long for Caroline's visit to the veterinarian. Gorgeous George, a beautiful Huskie, had come to court, and we were expecting. Before Fred and Mollie could take up residence in their new home, Caroline gave birth, in the chicken house, to a brood of nine.

I watched as Caroline birthed her young. She meticulously cleaned and examined each new arrival and required no help or advice from me.

For the next two weeks, I watched Caroline tirelessly nurse her babies. She was so vigilant in her efforts that she developed sores from lying too long. Later, she began to leave her frequently sleeping flock and take exercise with the other dogs.

As her pups grew, Caroline instinctively knew when they were ready to wean and left her place by their side. Her breasts, hanging low, became painfully engorged with milk. During this period, she kept watch over her yelping young from a distance.

After her milk stopped flowing, Caroline again laid with her puppies.

As I watched Caroline exhausted and still nursing, looking deprived herself, I related it to the feeling I have after a particularly exhausting and demanding week with my patients. I was reminded of a statement by Dr. Deckert, a medical school psychiatry professor, that, "In medicine, one sometimes feels one is wearing a coat lined with rows of nipples."

Through all of Caroline's efforts, Gorgeous George would occasionally come to call. He lazed about being no help at all. I felt like reporting him for overdue child-support.

FRED

After the winter birthing, the spring brought new homes for Caroline's puppies, and new chickens joined Fred and Mollie in the poultry yard. That summer, my flock dwindled as they flew out, becoming dog food, and the hawks and owls flew into the pen for dinner. I lost Mollie that summer, but Fred grew into a powerful strutting cock, with tail and wing feathers of black and emerald laced with gold.

Fred's bugle heralded each rising sun. In the chicken yard, Fred crowed and challenged the world as he proudly strutted his plumage, until the advent of Rodney. Rodney, a young rooster, was going through puberty. His voice was changing. He began to spar with Fred for territory. One morning, I found Fred dead. I guess Rodney won. Fred was a proud cock. Maybe that was the lesson. Pride has an early death.

RODNEY

One morning, engrossed in my writing, I was startled from my reverie by Rodney's agitated crow. I thought maybe he was scaring off the snake that gobbled up Blackie's first nesting eggs. Afraid to leave the nest, she had diligently been sitting a new batch for more than two weeks.

Hoe in hand, I charged out to the chicken house to kill the varmint. Instead, I was greeted by a still sitting hen and a bright-eyed freshly hatched chick, looking just like mom. Rodney had been crowing because he was a new papa.

I returned to the house and mused, "Isn't it just like a man?" Rodney was still out there crowing his head off as if he'd done the work, while Blackie silently sat.

THE AVIARY

To halt the attrition of my fowl population, I decided to build an aviary, also known as putting a lid on my chicken pen.

When I was in medical school and my oldest son Billy was a small child, I became very depressed and overwhelmed, and I neglected his parakeet, Chester. Chester died. For twenty-five years I carried guilt for that bird's neglect. No longer shrouded by depression, my building of the aviary felt like my atonement for the death of the parakeet. In therapy with patients and in my own process, I am frequently amazed how the emotional dots are connected and defused.

After completing my aviary, in addition to the emotional resolution, I surveyed my handiwork and concluded it surely had to be the fanciest chicken pen in Oklahoma county. After all my years of training and accomplishments, I reflected on the satisfaction I derived from such a laborious and menial task as putting a lid on my chicken pen.

BEN

When my black Labrador, Ben, was one year old, he would not leave my laundry alone. When Ben was loose and it was laundry day, some of my wash would wind up in the front yard.

I would look out the window and see that big black dog reared on his hind legs, stretching to get the one piece he desired. No matter whether I praised or punished, Ben continued to pull my laundry off the line. Eventually on laundry day, as much as I disliked to, I had to chain Ben.

The same thing happened with my children. No, I did not chain them, even though at times I liked the idea. Sometimes their behaviors were unacceptable, and positive and negative reinforcement failed. Then I resorted to hard-line consequences, also known as "tough love." Giving tough love was often painful for me and them, but I loved them enough to expend the energy to do what I knew was in their best interest.

To keep the laundry clean, sometimes I had to do things I didn't like for Ben and my children.

GRETA

My dogs, the castoffs of others, have such good souls and give me bountiful love.

Greta, a brindle pit bull, came to the farm and me as a starving and battered soul. In time, her body grew strong and muscular, and her spirit became happy and peaceful.

One morning, I found Greta curled in her favorite spot in the dog house, dead from a snake bite. The day before she had been vibrant, healthy, happy, and alive.

I am so glad I had my time with Greta. We often talked together, and as I stroked her head she would look lovingly into my eyes. Of all my dogs that are no longer earthbound, I miss Greta the most, and I continue to look for her in each new dog that comes to the farm.

TIZZY

At the death of his mother, my friend David's only inheritance was his mother's pet, Tizzy, an eight-year-old miniature Yorkshire terrier.

Following her owner's death, Tizzy went into mourning, and David was concerned she might also die.

Hoping Tizzy might respond to a feminine owner, David brought her to me and, after a few weeks in my home, her appetite returned. On my arriving home from work, with the origins of her name apparent, Tizzy bounces with glee and, at night, she curls up and sleeps with me. Tizzy has stolen my heart.

When David visits, he talks to Tizzy. Often, with multiple colorful names, he cusses and discusses her various attributes, but I know he is all bluff and bluster. Tizzy has him in her paw.

When I am home, Tizzy loves to lie quietly touching me. She is never agitated, barking, or demanding. She has a gentle, quiet spirit. She asks only to be, and on that topic she is my teacher.

OTTO

Otto needed a new home. Otto was an eight-month-old papered and pedigreed German rottweiler. At the time of his arrival into my country menagerie of dogs, he held the unique position of being the youngest and biggest. I later called him my "bouncing baby boy."

Having been a house dog, Otto's first night on the farm was made memorable by visions of his large head and paws as seen through the windows and door. Shades of Marmaduke.

I loved to watch Otto frolic and play with the other dogs, all except Sam. Sam, a huskie mix that I had brought from Alaska, was the top dog on the hill, and he early established his status with his towering younger brother.

Otto loved to bark and bounce around the chicken pen, where Rodney, safe inside, taunted and teased him.

Best of all, I enjoyed Otto as he followed me about, ever watchful and protective. As I worked on my building projects, Otto found a shady spot and kept me company. We had frequent conversations, and I often patted his big lovable head. Otto, my bouncing baby boy, had a heart of gold and teeth of steel, like several people I know.

After Otto had been with me about a year, he was absent three days. On the fourth day, I found a remnant of his hide that one of the dogs had carried into the yard. I suppose he tangled with a bobcat, poisonous reptile, or human. Freedom and the farm has its price.

I miss Otto's smiling mug. Otto lived life with gusto. He constantly played and explored, and nothing escaped his interest. Frequently on my returning home and opening the car door, he would poke his big head inside to greet me. He loved to chase the lawnmower and chickens, and before I put a lid on the chicken pen, I retrieved many a chicken from the clutches of his jaws. My other dogs miss his playfulness, and Sam misses his sparring partner.

Otto was a teacher for me. He definitely enjoyed each day of his all-too-short life. I suspect he is in heaven right now, licking God in the face. If we all lived each day with Otto's zest, when death came, we would know we had lived.

Pets are wise teachers with divine connections. I usually ask my patients if they have pets, because pets are important in our often lonely lives. They, unlike most humans, love us unconditionally.

CHAPTER THREE

Society's Foibles

IN THE FOIBLES OF OUR SOCIETY, we are often disconnected from our earth and our primal essence. To secure the safety of the planet and to reclaim our true Selves, we have many lessons to learn.

For example, we have created an instant and disposable society that pollutes the earth and squanders her resources. We have created a plastic and cellophane existence, with instant food, instant houses, and instant messaging. In doing so, we have estranged ourselves from the substance of life, such as preparing our food, building our homes, and working with wood, metal, and the earth. The lifestyle of instant gratification is devoid of communion with ourselves and our environment.

In contrast, I was reared in rural Oklahoma, lived five years in Alaska, and spent several months in the rugged and sparsely populated Alaskan Bush. In these environments, I lived close to the earth, my rhythms moved with hers and, as the seasons waxed and waned, I harvested her bounty.

Her bounty includes Alaskan blueberries. When autumn came, I hunkered down on the forest floor and gathered the succulent berries, all the while hoping a bear wasn't interested in the same patch. When winter arrived and the earth was snow-laden, I baked blueberry pies and muffins and, each time I removed the fragrant pastries from the oven, I resavored my days of berry picking.

When I contrast these poignant memories with rolling a cart down the supermarket aisle and picking berries out of a freezer case, everything is lost. I am saddened when I realize many people have never picked berries, harvested their food, or known this healing and life sustaining communion with the earth.

In psychiatry, there was a time when hospitalized patients' treatments included tending gardens and farm animals. Now, they are warehoused in large buildings, akin to prisons, with little earth contact. Perhaps we could empty a few mental wards if patients were outside harvesting her bounty and allowing the earth to aid in their healing.

On my Oklahoma farm, I find peace and satisfaction in living close to the land, preparing a meal from food I grew in my garden, hanging laundry on a clothesline, and building my own home. On the farm, I synchronize my life with the wind, sun, and rain, with the earth's ebb and flow, and my connection with the earth restores my soul.

THE SACRED

In spiritual teachings, I read that the sacred is in the ordinary, so I look for and find the sacred in my daily life.

For instance, food preparation for oneself and others is a sacred and loving act, and this sacrament extends to the utensils in which we prepare and store food. For such purposes, I collect an odd assortment of antique glassware, from which I receive much visual and tactile pleasure. My glassware includes Depression— green measuring cups and mixing bowls and Fire King casserole dishes with raised floral patterns. I have refrigerator containers of all colors and shapes, plus pint, quart, and half-gallon jars with glass lids and wire latches. All of these containers are made of thick heavy glass. They have substance. They were made to endure.

Similarly, I daily use my collection of antique German, French, Czechoslovakian, and Austrian china. Food tastes better and nourishes my soul when served on such beauty.

In contrast, the sacredness of food preparation is diminished by the use of plastic or disposable kitchenware. These products are transient, insubstantial, of no consequence. As I stock my kitchen shelves, I receive pleasure as I view and hold each object. Eventually I will share this collection with my daughter, daughter-in-law, and granddaughters. These objects speak to me of home, family, beauty, and my Grandmother Ollie. They tell of a time when the pace of life was slower and women and children talked together as they stood at the kitchen sink, washed, and dried dishes.

This image is contrasted to a dishwasher. Certainly, I have had dishwashers. They serve me well as storage bins. Machines have robbed us of our communion with our environment. In our haste to "save time," whatever that means, we overlook the sacred.

Along similar lines, machines have also become our society's favored form of "communication." With the Internet, e-mail, voice mail, and fax, machines are often the intermediary between ourselves and others. We too infrequently talk eyeball to eyeball.

Our days are becoming devoid of the sight, smell, sound, and touch of another human being. This sensory feast is replaced by fingertips on a keyboard. However, I still believe in buying stamps, writing notes by hand, and talking person to person. In connecting on a more personal plane, we have the opportunity to commune soul to soul.

We live in a lonely time, and part of the problem is that machines have become our intermediary between each other and our world. Every human being is a manifestation of Divine Presence and needs to be seen, heard, touched, and smelled. My dentist certainly has much to learn about the needs of the human spirit. He is young and skilled and has a big, new office full of machines. He treats two, three, or more patients at one time. He hops back and forth between us. I feel like an open mouth on an assembly line. He has overhead televisions in each room, for his patients to watch while he hops. If I ask a question, he usually selects a tape, and I am supposed to view the answer on television. I really just want him to talk to me. I want to connect with him and build trust before he does a root canal or fills a cavity in my all too vulnerable mouth. I know he is young and paying for lots of machines, but we all need to be treated like human beings instead of open mouths on a conveyor belt.

In our society's affair with machines, plastic, and cellophane, we abandon our communion with the earth, each other, and ourselves.

PIMPS

Pimps are varied and abundant in our society. I live on a 144-acre farm, thirty miles outside of Oklahoma City. As I travel between work and home, I observe large parcels of farm land cut into five-acre tracts and sold as "country living." On the realty signs, I often see one individual's name. I consider him a white-collar pimp.

Pimps and prostitution have been part of the human experience and viewed with contempt and scorn since Biblical days, but we often raise to high public esteem those individuals called "land developers," also known as "pimps of the earth."

Prostitution comes in all forms. We prostitute our souls for money and prestige, our values to conform to the norm, our children to satisfy our egos, and the earth in the name of progress.

Many spiritual paths revere God in every living form, be it human, animal, air, water, or a blade of grass. Their followers are not seduced by outward "progress." They value inward growth. Individuals who live by such beliefs know that the soul cannot find happiness in the illusions of the material world. They believe spiritual poverty and not material lack is the cause of all human suffering. Our society has much to learn.[1]

A Bygone Era

Growing up in the fifties, I watched the Perry Como and Dinah Shore shows, the Hit Parade, and feel-good movies. These movies and music were about families, children, animals, hope, dignity, and courage. In that era, the feelings of compassion, love, and respect were honored.

Then came the sixties, seventies, and eighties, and cynicism prevailed.

Now, movies are about sex, rape, and murder, and human dignity and courage are rare commodities. I find no social worth in these movies, which focus on societal depravation rather than values to which society needs to aspire.

There is an old Barbara Stanwyck and Gary Cooper movie set in the Depression. The movie is about a man who called himself John Doe. He spoke to the people of their worth and how their thoughts and actions could change the world. In the movie, John Doe Societies sprang up, and people worked together to help themselves and their families and communities.

I wonder what would happen if several times in one month all the television networks showed only that movie? Even if the programming didn't sell as many cars or boxes of soap, I wonder if national violence would decrease that month? I wonder what would happen if John Doe Societies sprang up across America and people banded together for the common good without regard to race, religion, or economic status?

I was again reminded of earlier times and values when en route to Washington, D.C., to visit my son Billy. I was intrigued by and stared at an African-American man wearing a vintage pork-pie hat. On apologizing for my staring, I met Eric. In our conversation, I discovered Eric was the lead singer of a D.C. band, and he invited Billy and me to his band's performance at a local club. The band was comprised of a clarinet and bass player, guitarist, saxophonist, pianist, drummer, and Eric. The music was of a bygone era of the Cotton Club and Savoy. The dancers performed the Jitterbug and Lindy Hop. They wore short skirts, suspenders, and saddle oxfords. The music made me feel good, had an identifiable beat, and I understood the words. I enjoy watching old movies with Lena Horne and the Cotton Club and, for one D.C. night, I experienced the beauty of that bygone era. Our society too often cherishes the newest gadget, music, or movie, but the first half of the twentieth century has lessons for this new age.

DIFFERENT DRAPERIES

I once facilitated a group in which a member said, "We all live in the same house, just with different draperies," and I was struck by the wisdom in that statement. I thought of how often we exclude individuals and experiences from our lives because we think they are different or beneath us. I was also reminded of this when shopping with my friend and neighbor, Jean Anne, at her favorite thrift store.

As we entered the store, I initially perused the merchandise and saw nothing of interest but, as I watched Jean Anne skillfully rummage through the stacks, I began to look more closely. Slowly, there emerged to my awareness many lovely and usable items.

Being hesitant, I did not open a chest-of-drawers, but Jean Anne opened each drawer and pulled out scarves for my examination. I chose three, with my favorite being a beige Italian print for nineteen cents.

Then, I found the fabric shelves and selected colorful pieces I could make into pillow cases.

One of Jean Anne's finds, and for twenty-five cents my most unique purchase, was a 1942 "Vogue's Book of Smart Dressmaking."

After looking through the castoffs of others, I purchased two books, three scarves, and four pieces of fabric, for a total of four dollars. My thrift store trip was a reminder of how often I, and others, overlook or cast aside lovely and worthy items and people.

Along similar lines, we often exclude individuals because of their sexual preference. I observed a celebration of our human differences when I visited Dupont Circle, located near my son Billy's law school apartment in Washington, D.C. Apparently, a large gay community resides near Dupont Circle, and I enjoyed observing this community's openness and freedom. Without fear of censorship, gay couples walked holding hands and openly showing affection. There was an atmosphere of acceptance. Spring was in bloom. Couples walked their dogs, bought flowers from street vendors, and ate in outdoor cafes. Laughter and chatter permeated the air.

I applaud all who follow their inner truth and live in peace and harmony with themselves and others or, as my friend Kevin tells people regarding the topic of same sex relationships, "If it's your cup of tea, drink it good." As for me, I celebrate our human differences, and perhaps eventually society as a whole can do the same.

Because of a difference in the color of skin or country of origin, members of our society often discriminate against and are hostile toward others they view as "different." What a tragedy.

I once thought, "If I came back in another life, I'd like to be an African-American NBA basketball player, like Michael Jordan, Tim Duncan, or Alan Iverson. I'd like to soar to the hoop, suspended in space and time."

Then, I stopped and remembered the plight of the African-American male in our society. I do not know what it feels like to be in his skin and to see the world through his eyes. How is he treated? Why does he so frequently become addicted or incarcerated? Why does he die so young?

My heart cries for him. What degradation does he endure climbing out of the mire of prejudice in our society?

After I stopped and thought about it, I don't know about another lifetime, but for this one, I will just sit back and applaud African-American male basketball players, as they soar to the hoop. This is their time and their space.

On further examination of our society's racial issues, Maze's Frankie Beverly gets down and funky as he sings in a throaty, gravelly voice "Color Blind."

We've been judging people by color,
Maybe we should all be color blind.
What I want to know is what color have you colored peace?
What color is harmony?
What color have you colored peace?
What color is harmony?
...can't judge a book by its cover
...what are we doing but just that.
We've been judging people by their color.
Love ain't got no color, that's a fact.

What color have you colored peace, love, and harmony?

I was reminded of Maze's song on a visit to the Smithsonian. The museum exhibited a black and white photographic collection by Chester Higgins, Jr., "The Spirit of the People," which depicted the African people from Harlem to Guiana. The exhibit featured pictures of people of all ages engaged in all types of activities. There were the eyes and faces of the young and old, of the sad and glad, and of those deep in thought, but the picture that most spoke to me was of an African Muslim woman wearing a white scarf and veil, exposing only the eyes, the most incredible eyes, the eyes of the soul. Those eyes saw and understood all. They looked deep within me, and we were one and the same. We get so caught up in the color of skin, but if we just looked at the eyes, we would know we were all one and the same, the same "Spirit of the People."

We often exclude people from our life experience because of their profession. My friend Jean Anne's husband, Louis, has been a truck driver for thirty years. When he is home, Jean Anne and Louis often invite me and others to the family dinner table. There I listen to Louis and his driver friends regale us with their trucking stories. However, beneath the humor, I hear the long lonely times cooped up in that twenty-four-hour moving cubicle of a freightliner going coast to coast on that endless white-lined asphalt. The drivers run, as they call it, in pairs, with one sleeping and the other driving. They talk of their late night deliveries in the often-dangerous downtowns of our cities. The drivers talk of little sleep, cold food, and lots of coffee. They have a jargon all their own. They are kind of like modern day cowboys, and the ones I've met have hearts as big as all outdoors.

Louis's driver friend, David, once related an experience that has always inspired him. He told of a trip many years before while he was delivering a load to Memphis, Tennessee. David stopped to ask a black man for directions. The man said, "My name is Red. Can I unload your truck?" As they became acquainted, Red asked David if it was alright to call him "Youngen," and David said, "Yeah." Red told David he lived in Mississippi with his wife and four children. Each morning, Red hitchhiked to Memphis to unload trucks. David asked, "Wasn't it hard to get a ride?" Red responded, "No, everybody knows me and that I live by the Word." Red said, "Times are hard for black people in Mississippi ... nothing's changed." In spite of it all, Red's wife had never worked out of the home, and Red had "put two of his kids through college." Years later, when David was sleeping in a truck, waiting to be unloaded, he heard someone knocking on the truck and saying, "Hey Youngen, you in there?"

There was Red. Red was the "yard guy" or manager of the large truck yard and, that day, while David rested, Red's crew unloaded David's truck at no charge. As they renewed their friendship, David asked Red how he had made his way. Red replied, "No matter how bad things got, I always looked to the Scripture and, if a man does that and works hard, everything is going to work out right."

Before you exclude someone from your life experience because of their skin color, profession, or sexual preference, remember, "We all live in the same house, just with different draperies."

PAPERWORK

The complexity of our societal structure and the nonsense this structure propagates is exemplified by its forms and paperwork. Our society spawns forms like Jeffrey's guppies spawn babies, willy-nilly and profusely. Required information forms are so intrusive, I am amazed they don't ask for our underwear size. Once, with a form to work for a government agency, I was required to have a medical examination of every orifice of my body. I felt like a horse at an auction having my teeth examined. In this age of computers, surely there is a giant computer in the sky that has all of my, and your, vital statistics duly recorded for posterity. That is one of the few machines I would vote for, then I wouldn't have to fill out another dang form.

Once, after receiving forms that recorded the theft of my two electrical generators, I was amused as I filed the folder entitled "Theft" right behind taxes. At the time of the theft, I was consoled when the police officer said I could file the personal loss as a tax deduction. Later I called my accountant and was told this was true only if the theft was ten percent of my yearly net income. In other words, the thieves have to steal more, or one thief or another is going to take me to the cleaners.

I consider insurance companies and their entwined shell game of paperwork another form of legalized theft and insanity. The mountain of paperwork that insurance companies and state and federal health care agencies proliferate could fell many a forest. The situation with health care insurance is so insane the companies set the fee schedules (also called price fixing), dictate who the patient will see for services, where they will be seen, how long they will be seen, and what medications they will receive. This is all decided with little or no medical education or regard for the patient's preferences or welfare.

I was once stunned when told one state health care agency no longer reimbursed psychiatrists for medication management of a large segment of the chronically mentally ill and disabled. As one psychologist jokingly stated, "What are we supposed to treat them with, M&Ms?"

I have wondered, with the insanity on the part of insurance companies, state and federal health care agencies, if they should be treated with a good antipsychotic like Thorazine, Mellaril, or Haldol. If an individual acted with the insanity or deceit of insurance companies and governmental agencies, the individual would be imprisoned or hospitalized and the key thrown away.

Along such lines, my friend Lucas commented on governmental vagaries as he railed at the "energy saver" on his hot water heater, which resulted in mid-point lukewarm showers, and the "water saver" on his toilet requiring "five flushes" to clear the bowl. He concluded, "The government shouldn't be in my bathroom."

Similarly, work-related injuries often get buried in paperwork and defrauded by insurance companies. Following an on-the-job injury, I once accompanied David to a number of doctor appointments. At those visits I observed extremely unethical behavior on the part of two physicians. David was required by employee regulations to see physicians dictated by the employer's insurance company. When I asked to join David to hear the results of his studies, twice the physician's staff asked if I was an attorney? After those questions, I said, "No," and did not bother to inform them I was a physician. I witnessed two physicians lie regarding the results of MRI reports. They each, independently, told my friend the results were "normal."

I had reviewed the report and knew the results were clearly abnormal, and the results of the MRI determined the type of care David received and if he would be compensated for the job-sustained injury.

It is a sad commentary when insurance companies determine the quality of medical care, or lack thereof, of work-related injuries, and these companies are aided and abetted by workmen's compensation laws and the mountain of paperwork these laws generate.

Neighbors

One day my neighbor Jean Anne brought me a dozen eggs she had just gathered from her hens. What a treat. It harkened to the days of my Grandmother Ollie, her Arkansas home, and her country values. The following morning as I relished the golden scrambled mounds, I thought fondly of my neighbor's kindness. You know, rural America still exists, and whether you are a rural or an urban dweller, exchanging homegrown or prepared goods can be a thing of the present.

We can, and many have, revive the practice of sewing, baking, and growing food for our families, friends, and neighbors. One summer my garden was abundant, and I enjoyed giving away squash, green beans, and okra. The following winter, on a visit to my veterinarian, he commented how much he had enjoyed the squash I gave him. Each of us can spread joy by extending a little neighborly kindness.

On the subject of neighbors, have you ever noticed some neighborhoods seem to compete for the prize of who has the biggest, most expensive house? Some neighborhoods are so exclusive that one has to enter through guards or electronic gates. Such neighborhoods seem to scream, "We have money. We are the elite. Keep out."

For me these neighborhoods often seem like sterile and lifeless forms of conspicuous consumption, building bigger and better piles of rock. What happened to homey, comfortable, and cozy? In some of these neighborhoods, the houses look as though the occupants would have to wear starched underwear to bed. Some of the houses are more groomed and pedicured than their occupants. Sometimes I think these neighborhoods are a form of prison, with the occupants held hostage by their egos.

I have often mused on local exclusive neighborhoods entitled "Oaktree," "Oakdale," and "Oakmont." I often thought of hoisting a sign over the entrance to my farm entitled "More Oaks - Black Jack Acres."

I once had a man describe the definition of success in his affluent neighborhood as living in a "cookie cutter house." He described his neighborhood's dictum that he send his children to college, then graduate school. The dictum further held that his children would then marry, have children, and all come home to the same "cookie cutter house" for Thanksgiving and Christmas. He felt like he was locked in a living death. To reside within such narrow societal confines is like living in a straitjacket that shrivels the soul.

Emotional healing requires unlacing oneself and opening the doors of one's mind. We often live in prisons imposed by our minds, our rearing, and our culture. Only we can unlace our straitjackets and open our prison doors.

THE SCOREBOARD

Thrown into a spiral of self-doubt, a successful businessman related to me the decline in his business. He developed his business from his creative and spiritual self. Later the business took on a life of its own and engulfed him. After the business monster spewed him out, the monster consumed itself, and the man became reacquainted with himself and his loves, passions, and God. Now the man is the artist in residence in his life and is redefining his work as an expression of his creative and spiritual self. We can all choose to be free of the monsters created by our egos and be our own artist in residence.

Likewise, after spending a number of months in intense emotional upheaval another businessman remarked, "I am an overachiever and overachievers keep score, and all I am doing in my healing does not show up in the score box."

His comment reflected his lack of putting business on his books and dollars in his bank account. We discussed the fact that our society often focuses on numbers instead of people and on the external rather than the internal. To the scoreboard, I suggested a load of buckshot. To society, I suggested a rearrangement of priorities, because God doesn't keep score that way.

THE LINES

My friend Janice once exclaimed, "I've colored in the lines all my life. I'm tired of it." We are a "color in the lines" society. Our rigid drive for perfection of body, mind, mate, child, pet, house, and car keeps us in a frenzy coloring in the lines. We color-coordinate our lives, trying to keep up with this year's set of colors and lines. Heaven forbid we don't match this year's fashion or our lines are a little smudged or blurred. In the sixties, we burned girdles and bras and stepped outside society's lines, but it seems we have cinched up again. I encourage you to throw away your straight edges, rulers, and blinders. Open your eyes. Open your mind. Color outside your lines.

◎ ◎ ◎

The foibles of society are our teachers. However, society is comprised of individuals. When each individual aspires to their highest Self in body, mind, and spirit, society will be elevated. The only person we can change is ourselves. When you are disturbed about society, look within. Change who you can. You.

CHAPTER FOUR

Simplify

OUR SOCIETY SEEMS TO GLORIFY IN COMPLICATING LIFE with more bells and whistles. In reading revered ancient teachings, the repeated message is to simplify.

I certainly had my turn at conspicuous consumption, including the big house replete with expensive furniture, rugs, crystal, and china, but there I found no peace.

Each level of my healing has required me to release more of my physical and emotional baggage. Today, I find peace on my farm living in a simple home that I built myself, for I have learned that "less is more" and "enough is enough," and it's best to just plain "keep it simple."

I learned much about simplifying my life in my sojourn in the Alaskan Bush. There I lived in a log home, with electricity, propane for cooking, and a wood stove for heat. I had no indoor plumbing. I hauled water and had an outhouse for necessities. Believe me, at twenty below, one makes quick night relief trips.

In the Bush, warm clothes and food, shelter, and a hot bath were premium commodities. With no plumbing, water was heated in a large pot on the stove, and bathing often consisted of a dish pan of hot water. Simple amenities are taken for granted in our society. We rush in all directions in our pursuit of toys, activities, and possessions, believing they will provide the ultimate "Aha." Today, I find pleasure in warm food, clean comfortable clothes, indoor plumbing, and bathing in lots of hot water. The ancients taught that the sacred is in the ordinary and, in the sacred, one knows bliss.

On returning to Oklahoma, my Alaskan lessons on simplicity served me well. I had learned one needs very little to live a peaceful and rich life. In Alaska, I saw simple homes of all descriptions built by their owners. I savored visiting those self-built homes, for the builders' imaginations, ingenuity, and unique creations delighted me.

In comparison, I drive through the Oklahoma countryside and observe the overnight appearance of single- and double-wide trailer houses that have sprouted like mushrooms or see new houses assembled instantly, with prefab and synthetic materials, similar to and just about as flavorful as instant pudding. Too often these houses are built for monetary expediency, with little or no emotional investment by the builder and no direct labor by the new homeowner.

My favorite uncle, Uncle Fred, was a carpenter of the old school, who meticulously built homes from scratch. As a child, I spent hours watching Uncle Fred measure, saw, and nail with his strong hands that had many parts of fingers missing from encounters with saws. Even with missing portions of digits, Uncle Fred was a fine craftsman.

I had wanted to build my own home since childhood, but I felt intimidated by this seemingly masculine domain.

However, while in Alaska, I saw a seventy-six-year-old woman splitting logs with an axe. She became my role model. I was determined that as I advanced in years I would be equally self-sufficient. To accomplish this goal, I decided that if I built my own home I could also repair it. Therefore, I wouldn't be afraid of being stranded alone without enough money or "a man." So, through this line of reasoning, I became one woman with a hammer, who built her own home board by board and nail by nail. My home isn't big or fancy, and I don't have Uncle Fred's skills. But what I lacked in craftsmanship, I made up for in heart and down-home flavor. Besides, I never liked instant pudding. I like the old double-boiler, stand-and-stir kind of pudding that is thick and luscious and has a few lumps, just like my house.

In planning to build my home, I read of many alternative building techniques, including rammed earth, rubber tire, cob, and hay bale houses. These techniques are very cost and energy efficient, and simple to build. I realize these building methods are labor intensive, but one can consider self-construction of one's home a good investment in one's physical and emotional health and a savings on gym fees.

In this instant society, it behooves us to consider more human-and earth-friendly alternatives. Before starting my home, I gained experience in building my generator/well house, chicken house, and barn. In my various construction projects, some of my building materials were discarded by others and included scrap rock, tires, and used boards and bricks. In this process, I took great delight in collecting and making creative use of these materials, and often the use of these building ma-

terials was a lot like quilting in which one takes seemingly use-
less bits, scraps, and shapes of fabric and makes a beautiful,
usable whole.

At times, my building technique also drew on my quilting
skills. Being an inexperienced carpenter, I found I had unexpected gaps and spaces. With a little quilting, however, I struc-
turally and cosmetically made corrections.

In this age of perfectionism and "How To" books, I find it
pleasant to realize there is more than one "right way," and my
way can consist of a little quilting.

Besides learning to saw, hammer, and drill in preparing to
build my home, I read much about energy and heat conservation and producing my own electricity "off the grid." I decided
to use a combination of solar power, generators, and possibly
fuel cells. On moving to the farm, I used a generator as my
only electrical source and streamlined my life to use as little
as possible of that energy called electricity. I simplified my few
electrical needs to lights and power to run the water pump. As
for the "conveniences," I use a propane stove and refrigerator
and, for additional sources of light, I use candles and kerosene
lamps. I have a wood stove for heat and two antique flat irons
for ironing. I do not own a computer, and I rarely watch television. I refuse to be held hostage by society's conveniences and,
by proclaiming my freedom from the electric company, I never
have to worry about the "power" going off.

However, without the convenience of a washer and dryer, I
had to adapt. To avoid the dreaded laundromat and like a true
frontier woman, I often wash my laundry by hand and hang it
on the clothesline. I find that I enjoy this simple task. It is good

exercise, my clothes get clean, and I have a personal relationship with my clothes, rather than a machine.

Often as I hang my laundry on the clothesline, I watch the sun shine on the red-brown plaster-swirled earth covering the hay bale walls of my generator/well house. I feel pride in this building that might look rough and crude to others. My children and I built that generator/well house, and I consider it a work of art.

As a child and young adult, I thought pleasure and fulfillment would come from college graduation and the purchase of expensive houses, cars, and clothes, but I was wrong. Through my healing, my life's evolution has been one of increasing simplicity. I now know pleasure and fulfillment come from the simplest things, like hanging laundry on a clothesline, baking a pie, or watching the sun reflect from the walls of my generator/well house.

CENTRAL HEAT AND AIR

My simple home is placed on the land for the sun, breezes, view, and protection from winter's north winds. My home's central heat is a wood stove in the center of the living room, with a propane backup. In Alaska, I enjoyed cutting and stacking wood and using a wood stove. On my farm, my main crop is scrub brush. As I clear the overgrowth, I provide wood for the winter, and my body enjoys the exercise and power it feels in performing this labor of love.

In the Alaskan summers, I did not live in an air-conditioned bubble. My home was open to nature. On returning to Oklahoma, my sources of "air-conditioning" are open windows, shade trees, breezes, and fans. In nature's wisdom, sweat cools and purifies the body.

My old-fashioned form of central heat and air restores me to balance and harmony with my environment and grounds me in the primal essence of my being.

During hot Oklahoma summers, I drive down the road in my old brown truck with open windows. As I drive, I see closed air-conditioned houses and cars. In treating the environment as an enemy, the occupants miss the smells of plowed fields and pastures with freshly mowed grass. They miss the welcome breeze on bare skin and the sound of crickets in the blazing sun.

Nature is a blessing and a teacher. I feel sad that we often treat her as an adversary and pack ourselves away in air-conditioned boxes. From the boxes, we can't smell, hear, or feel her gifts.

BE YOURSELF

In our pursuit of society's illusions, we often complicate our lives, delete the sacred, and lose ourselves in the process. In the ancient teachings of the "Tao Te Ching," written approximately 550-479 B.C., the old master states:

In dwelling, live close to the ground.
In thinking, keep to the simple.
In conflict, be fair and generous.
In governing, don't try to control.
In work, do what you enjoy.
In family life, be completely present.

When you are content to be simply yourself and don't compare or compete, everybody will respect you.[2]

CHAPTER FIVE

Wisdom

WE IN THE WESTERN WORLD often live in the illusion that wisdom and education come primarily from books and schools. I have learned more in my healing journey than I ever learned in school.

I know people with deep wisdom who cannot read or write. I hear people with "poor" diction render blinding insight into my life and the lives of others. People from all walks of life teach me in the most unexpected ways, and I am awed by their brilliance.

There is much to be gained from books and schools. However, the printed word and educational institutions can also be a source of confusion. I have heard it said, "In seeking knowledge much is acquired, in seeking wisdom much is discarded."

I often work with highly educated people. They come to me with their lives in a tangle and their heads filled with a myriad of facts and theories. With lives driven by external goals and minds jumbled with intellectual minutia, their truth is denied them.

In healing, they look deep within themselves and claim their truth and discard layers of facts and theories that are inconsistent with and irrelevant to their truth. In this process, they become calm and centered and travel from knowledge to wisdom.

Our society seems to glorify in intellectual trivia, almost to the point of perpetual mental masturbation, and this is done under the guise of "knowledge." Anyone can read a book and regurgitate its contents, but the wise discern whether the book's meaning has value.

Teachers

I have been told, "When the student is ready, the teacher appears." I believe we are all teachers; some just teach by negative example. I believe we are all students; some are just more willing to learn than others.

In my life, I found I could not receive the lessons until I had prepared myself to become the student. For so long, because of pride, arrogance, and fear, I was not teachable. I thought only those with lofty educations or social status could teach me, but I was wrong.

I have found my teachers in country folks and their rural wisdom, in the faces and words of children, and in the supposedly "uneducated."

Oh, many of the educated and socially prominent have taught me, but sometimes they taught me what I did not want to become.

How does the student become ready? I suspect readiness comes most frequently through pain. When our answers aren't working, we become willing to open to all of life's teachers and lessons.

Wisdom's Price

In my healing, I have found wisdom's price to be high. The price is always pain.

For over twenty years, I have been friends with Mary. Mary is a physician with Bipolar Disorder, also known as Manic-Depressive Disorder. I have watched the ravages of Mary's illness batter her spirit and strip her of her profession, self-confidence, and hope.

At times, I feared Mary would choose death. Now, as she and I are both past fifty, I see her life has made her strong, serene, and wise. She has buffeted the storms of her illness and found peace in her family and church, and she is now sought for her wisdom.

Mary and I agree our wisdom had a high price, but I feel neither of us would change the women we became through its purchase.

LOOK WITHIN

Our planet abounds with God's messengers and teachers, but the greatest teacher lies within. I was reminded of this many years ago while visiting Texas' Big Bend State Park. While there, I found a biography on the then eighty-year-old Jewel Babb. Ms. Babb lived the latter portion of her life on the Texas-Mexico border. She grew up in the days of horse-pulled wagons and cattle roundups. She married, raised children, and in later years, discovered her healing powers. When her biography was written, she resided alone, living in a home without electricity or running water. There many sought her for her wisdom, her cures, and to learn her healing methods.

Since I read the book on this wise healing woman, I have remembered Ms. Babb's lessons. She said, "Television makes me sick. People who look at TV know what other people know.

I want to know what I know." Ms. Babb added, "If you go to church, you'll hear it how they tell it. But if you sit on a hill for fifteen years, with your animals and no one else, you learn a lot. It comes to you."[3]

As I live in solitude on my farm, I turn inward to my divine connection. With the Border Healing Woman as my guide, I have been sitting on my hill with my animals for several years, because I want to know what I know.

PART TWO

Changing Perspective

CHAPTER SIX

Positive Focus

HOW WE THINK ABOUT OR PERCEIVE OUR WORLD determines our feelings, actions, and health. Unfortunately, our media glorifies in the base, crass, and depraved, because fear sells newspapers, insurance, medicine, beauty products, and other goods ad infinitum. Fear and negativity make money, because when people are afraid, they can be led. For our personal healing and the healing of the planet, we must change our life's perspective. If one is centered in God, love, kindness, and looking for the positive in every life event, one reclaims one's power.

Our minds are powerful, and what we think we manifest. The concept that every thought we have and every word we utter contains energy to manifest itself has been put forth by spiritual teachers throughout time. In discussing the twelfth century's Hildegard of Bingen's spiritual remedies, Strehlow writes, "Every word is potent and powerful in our brains...A word can kill or heal; it can be a poison or a remedy...Positive thoughts deactivate negative energy and activate the healing power of our souls."[4] Likewise, Dr. David Hawkins writes, "Energy follows thought, or what is held in the mind tends to materialize."[5] To achieve our highest good and the highest good for all concerned, we must choose kind, loving, life-affirming thoughts, words, and actions.

Through the path of positive thought and many teachers and lessons, my life has been a journey inward toward love, light, and God. A prayer in the Hindu tradition begins, "May our ears hear the good, may our eyes see the good,"[6] and I have added, "May my mind seek the good." My healing required me to think of, listen for, and see the good in every person and life event.

Since our thoughts and words are energetically powerful, we must be selective about what we send out into the planetary energetic airways. In our society, we often function under the delusion that if we criticize someone, including ourselves, they will become or do what we think they ought to be or do. Just the opposite happens. We poison their spirits with thoughts and words that become self-fulfilling prophesies.

It is also said that what we energetically send out into the universe returns to us, or "What goes around, comes around." If we send out sarcasm, criticism, and negativity, we receive it back. It is like sending out a boomerang loaded with manure. Likewise, if we send out love, kindness, and acceptance, we get it back, often multiplied.

I like to acknowledge and thank those who send out positive energy and make my world a little brighter. For example, several years ago I was working in a rural clinic. One day as I received my change from my usual lunchtime cashier, I commented how cheerful she always looked. She replied, "When I feel myself getting down, I think I might as well be glad as sad."

In complimenting her on her positive attitude, she gifted me with her homespun wisdom.

Certainly, I do not wish one to deny one's feelings of sadness or grief; however, after those feelings are experienced and processed, one can choose to release them and affirm one's life lessons, or one can choose to remain stuck in a quagmire of self-pity and anger, continually repeating a litany of woes. I have seen individuals in the most dire circumstances look for and find the positive, spirit-affirming message within their situation, and from seeming ashes they bloom.

On the other hand, some people seem to delight in "ain't it awful" sessions. No matter how one works to refocus them toward positive thoughts, these individuals can always find the negative, and they seem determined to pull everyone into the mud with them.

I have heard it said, "If we focus on the problem, the problem increases and, if we focus on the solution, the solution increases." How we choose to think and act is our choice, but remember your thoughts and actions will determine your feelings. Would you rather be sad or glad?

If you choose to be glad and look for the positive, it can be found within any life event. Once, after a hard day's work, I came home to my farm and found thieves had come calling. They had cut a heavy metal chain and stolen both of my generators. I was without electricity.

I called 911 and the fellow asked if I wanted a police officer to come or could he take the report over the phone? He obviously preferred the latter and, of course, I preferred the former. Before my eyes, I wanted my theft appropriately and duly recorded.

Later, I called my neighbors and heard that someone else, a mile away, had also been robbed that day. Obviously, the theft was nothing personal.

I looked for the positive in this event and began to think of ways to operate without electricity. The main use of my generators was for my water pump and lights, but I was in no immediate need because I had candles and stored containers of water. I strongly considered constructing a windmill for pumping my water supply, thereby eliminating my need for electricity.

With those thoughts, I remembered that the last time I was without electricity, the month after my fiftieth birthday, my writer self was born. After silencing the world's chatter, who knows what else might birth from me? Life with God is always an adventure.

Whether our thoughts are positive or negative, our subconscious mind hears everything we say and think and manifests in our lives the messages it receives. Simply, we become what we think so, when I listen to my patients, I often take notes of their exact words and read back to them the words they tell themselves. They often call themselves "failures, impotent, fat, ugly, stupid." The list is endless of the abusive words people heap upon themselves.

If, for one year, you replaced each negative word you call yourself with the exact opposite, whether you believe it or not, you would be amazed how your life could be transformed. If you change the negative words to "success, virile, healthy, beautiful, and intelligent," your subconscious mind will hear and manifest these in your life. Our subconscious mind manifests what it hears. We become what we think. What do you choose to think?

As I focus on the positive in my life situations, I have learned that God has incredible timing and a wonderful sense of humor. One day, I attended a meeting and waxed eloquent on focusing on the positive. Later in the day, while at work, I received a call telling me there had been a grass fire on my farm and about fifty acres of underbrush had burned, barely missing my home, barn, and animals.

While driving home, I reflected on the fire which destroyed my childhood home when I was six. The fire had consumed all of my toys and clothes and left me and my family homeless. That night driving home, I said many prayers of gratitude, mused on God's timing, and could truly focus on the positive. My animals and belongings were safe, and I knew fire is nature's way of clearing and restoring the land and, afterward, the land flourishes.

When I arrived home, I was greeted by at least ten flashing fire trucks. I was told earlier there had been many more, plus helicopters and three television news stations. So much for the quiet and anonymity of the country.

In the dark, I viewed the damage. To make room for the fire trucks, small trees had been pulled out by the roots. The earth had been soft, with many trucks becoming stuck, leaving my yard crisscrossed by ruts and, with the weight of the trucks, there was the possible destruction of my septic system. All in all, I felt extremely calm and grateful.

The following day, I was reminded of the Chinese proverb, "Since my house burned, I have a better view of the moon." Even if the fire had consumed my belongings, I knew God would have shown me something for which to be grateful, for I am no longer a scared, lonely child. Yes, if my house had burned, I would have had a better view of the moon, even if it was a bit airy.

CHAPTER SEVEN

Aging : An Adventure

EACH YEAR OF OUR LIVES enriches our human becoming. However, a large segment of the American population approaches aging with fear. To fulfill our spiritual potential as we age, we must look beyond our physical forms and into the depths of our souls. For as we mature in wisdom, the beauty of our souls far outshines our earthly shells.

As I approached my maturation with vigor, I refused to be fettered by a number. On the morning of my fiftieth birthday I put my foot to a shovel in a ground-breaking ceremony and celebrated the adventure and knowledge that at fifty, with hammer in hand, I could build my own home. Those present included me, my dogs, and the birds.

One morning I found a wonderful metaphor for aging. Before going into the office that day, I picked the last of that season's blackberries. As I gathered the berries, I noticed how the most succulent berries were on the most brown-leafed, dried, and withered branches. Without looking closely, I could have easily missed them. I also noticed the largest branches with the most flamboyant leaves bore little or no fruit. How often we are seduced by the flamboyance of youth, often ignoring or even demeaning the aged, where the fruit lies.

Similarly, in the days of the Lexus and Mercedes, I drive an old brown truck which has dents, character, utility, and it gets me where I need to go. It's a lot like my body. With our society's focus on perfection—the new, the young, the creaseless faces, and bumpless thighs—there is not much room for my dents and character. Webster states that perfection is "The quality or state of being flawless." Let's get real. Perfection is an illusion. We are human beings, with all the wonderful flaws and irregularities of that condition.

As we age, we often demean ourselves with words or phrases such as "over the hill," whatever that means.

There are many hills in life. Those ups and downs are life.
There is the hill of a toddler, learning to walk.
There are the hills of puberty, adolescence, dating, and drugs.
There are the hills of marriage, first-born child, and children leaving home.
There is the hill of loss of a partner through death or divorce.
There are the hills of health, illness, recovering health, or death.
There are the emotional hills, dealing with the fractures and wounds of life.
When someone says, "I am over the hill, I just ask, "Which one?"

WOMEN AND AGING

As women age, our society tends to treat us as if we are produce on a shelf, with an expiration date. I revolt against the idea of treating women as perishable commodities. With age, women become richer human beings, with all the wisdom and grace born of time. We come into our own. Many of us make self-affirming choices about our life's journey and treat our age with reverence. Our fifties and beyond are our richest years, our wisdom years, and these years are to be savored.

Similarly, I once heard a friend say, "Antiques are alive, not just born out of the wrapper." What a lovely statement for furniture and people. In our society's endless quest for youth and "beauty," we often forget the beauty life renders the human form.

In my home, I enjoy using antiques of every description. These objects are beautiful and have character. Likewise, I relish observing and listening to people who have had long, full lives. Their experiences, pains, and joys have molded their human form and spirits into a work of art.

Contrast these to a new piece of furniture on a showroom floor or a seventeen-year-old beauty queen. They both may glitter and look pretty, but they have yet to fully develop their characters. Give me, any time, something or someone that has known life and wasn't "just born out of the wrapper."

OUR CHOICE

The quality of our life, our health, and how we age is largely our choice. Some cry that aging is determined by genetics, but genetics is only one factor. Science has amassed a large body of information documenting how exercise, nutrition, vitamins, hormonal replacement, alcohol, abused drugs, and smoking affect our bodies and minds and how we age.

Certainly, alcohol and abused drugs accelerate physical and mental deterioration. These can include anything from alcohol-related gastrointestinal cancers, liver disease, and dementia to the strokes and heart attacks of cocaine abuse to the mental deterioration with long-term marijuana usage.

From nicotine, tobacco, and smoking come cancers of the mouth, lungs, kidneys, and urinary bladder. Nicotine markedly accelerates vascular disease, resulting in strokes and heart attacks.

Research has well established that moderate exercise and healthy nutrition will improve physical health and increase longevity. Research has identified that healthy nutrition, exercise, continued mental activity, and vitamin therapy help prevent mental decline as we age. Some reports also show that post-menopausal estrogen replacement for women and possibly late-life testosterone replacement for men may also contribute to prolonged mental acuity.

Our health and how we age are largely our choice. I know my choice. What will you choose?

HUMOR

When all else fails, age with humor.

At one of my breast screening appointments, I sat for three hours with twenty-plus other women in a cold corridor as we awaited our mammograms, thermograms, and ultrasounds. Each of our upper bodies was covered with a loose "cape" held together in front by a clothespin. We each sat insulated in our own worlds, with only occasional passing conversation.

As I waited, I noticed a woman in her eighties, who walked with a cane and was about as round as she was tall. Due to her age, as she went from one exam to the next, a place was always made for her to sit. Once on sitting next to me on a fairly small chair, she fluffed out her ample body and humorously questioned out loud if the chair would support her bulk.

Once, on going down the aisle, the nurse commented, "I almost tripped you." Without skipping a beat, the octogenarian said, "Oh, you don't want to see that." A fall would obviously have exposed her upper body.

Minutes later after completing her exams and dressing, the elder lady stepped out of the restroom and, with a twinkle in her eye, announced to the group of unfamiliar women, "I just dropped my bra and prosthesis in the stool." The hall pealed with laughter. I doubled over, I laughed so hard. We all relaxed and liberally discussed some of the challenges of aging and our current compromising situation.

The lady was adorable. At eighty, our elder stateswoman with great aplomb shared with all of us waiting souls the humor of her body and actions. She reminded us to not take ourselves too seriously and to look for the humor as we age.

BIRTHINGS

Since I began writing this book and building my home, I have navigated several birthdays. During these years of my fifties, I have continued my inward travel and discovered what a blessing growing older is when, with each passing year, one takes part in birthing one's true Self. In this birthing, we strive to release ourselves from the bondage of this illusionary ego-driven world. In this ultimate of birthing journeys, we discover that our souls are immortal and only temporary occupants of a mortal form. In this quantum shift of perspective, we discover that we are souls having a human experience, and any sense of aging or death of this earthly vessel is of no consequence. What is of importance is how we live our lives. As we birth our divine Selves, we come to know that our purpose on the planet is to learn spiritual lessons and to help others in their spiritual journeys. As we shift our perspective from the earthly to the spiritual plane, the little inconveniences we experience in the aging process of this physical form are minor. For our life's purpose is for our souls to draw nearer to God.

CHAPTER EIGHT

Womanhood: A Changing View

I WAS BORN IN 1946. In the society of my rearing, a woman's life was confined to a relatively narrow box, but with the sixties, the view changed, especially in the arena of education.

In 1967, after three years of college, majoring in art history and philosophy, I quit school to become an "earth mother." By 1971, I was twenty-five and the mother of a three-year-old son. Any illusion I had of becoming a home-bound super-mom had vanished, and out of desperation, I returned to college. Thinking I might want to be employable in a shrinking job market, I planned a Ph.D. program in chemistry.

One evening during a chemistry lab, I was listening to a fraternity hot shot boast that he was a pre-med major. I casually asked him about the medical school entrance requirements, and I discovered that I had taken all the classes and made A's. Right then and there, I decided if that jerk could be a physician, so could I.

Now that is how God works in my life. Sometimes I receive these life changing moments of clarity from the most peculiar of sources. So, in the Fall of 1972, with several other women, wives, and mothers, I entered the University of Oklahoma

Medical School. We were the first wave of increasing numbers of women entering medicine and other previously male-dominated professions. We had to work hard for that entrance, and often the dues were very costly.

In medical school as in the society of my rearing, I felt being a woman was one step below nothing; however, I believed if I worked hard enough and was as good or better than any man, I might redeem myself from this fatal condition. That perception of myself was basically how I became a physician. On some level, I felt if I achieved that revered degree, surely then I would overcome this flaw of womanness, but not so in the society from which I issued.

Since my society of origin did not affirm me, I finally began to affirm myself for my womanness but, as with many seemingly obvious thoughts, I spent a long time beating myself before the idea came to me.

Eventually, I began to know the delightfulness of being a woman. We are resilient; we endure; we nurture; we suckle; we birth new life. In our later years, we have the wisdom born of time, living, and our connection with the earth. We flow with the earth and her rhythms. We are one with Mother Earth.

DR. DAN

One of my teachers in the value of my womanhood was Dr. Dan. By the time I met Dr. Dan, I had endured many dreaded yearly gynecological exams, been treated by a number of gynecologists of both genders, and felt like one of many cattle herded into a chute, a piece of meat going to market.

On the walls of Dr. Dan's waiting area, check-in room, and exam rooms hung pictures of babies he had delivered and funny woman-affirming sayings. As I waited on the examining table, in came Dr. Dan. He was kind and gentle. He talked to me. I felt valued as a woman and as a human being and that my health was important to him.

I sensed Dr. Dan chose obstetrics and gynecology because he revered new life and the procreative vessel of a woman's body.

As I grew older, my uterus was no longer needed for its re-productive function and, when it began to impair my health, Dr. Dan was my surgeon. Afterwards, I knew Dr. Dan valued my well-being and my womanhood and that my importance as a woman far exceeded my function as a walking womb.

PATRIARCHY

Unlike Dr. Dan, over the last three thousand years the world's social structure has been largely patriarchal and valued women for their capacity to bear children. Otherwise, women were largely denigrated and demeaned.[7] As human becomings, we must learn to cherish the feminine and masculine genders and celebrate their differences.

Our gender differences include the way we think and ap-proach problems. These differences are related to social condi-tioning and hormonal effects on the brain. The literature reports that testosterone changes the brain's axonal and dendritic devel-opment. Testosterone also changes the pre- and postneuronal synapses and the brain's neuronal distribution. Likewise, estro-gen has similar effects on the development of the feminine ner-vous system. Translated, men and women are wired differently.

God obviously created the gender differences to comple-
ment and balance each other, but for centuries our society
has proclaimed that the testosterone-dominated brain is
superior, and this mindset has affected every aspect of a
woman's life.

In our patriarchal society, men have often been the underlying force in many decisions about what women should be and
do and how they should look and, after thousands of years of
conditioning, women have often followed the patriarchal party
line. This conditioning is particularly apparent in the lengths
women will go to be considered attractive to and hopefully loved
and valued by the opposite sex.

FASHION

For the sake of "beauty" women have sacrificed their bodies
to the often male designer dominated fashion industry. At times,
the trappings of models on fashion runways resemble a freak
show. The fashion dictates of the fifties included permanents,
hair spray, high heels, cinched waists, and girdles. Heaven forbid
anything should jiggle or be out of place. Then came sack and
balloon dresses, bra burning, and elastic. Women could breathe.
This was followed by "professional dressing," with women looking like suited versions of men, replete with ties and pin stripes.
Now, fashion is again perpetrating its torture of the feminine
form and has revived the fifties and tight skirts and suit jackets,
spike heels, and girdles.

I once visited the New York Metropolitan Museum of Art's
exhibition of a twenty-five-year collection of a male Parisian designer. I was enlightened. Most of the clothes were designed for

flat-chested, prepubertal, anorexic females or males and were incongruent with an adult woman's form.

To wear these "fashionable designs," women have starved themselves and become frail and weak women. Wearing this attire in their malnourished state women look like survivors of a concentration camp. As women age in this malnourished state, they become senile and have stooped, wasted, osteoporotic bodies. The very nature of maturation into womanhood is the development of rounded breasts, hips, and thighs. The time has come for women to claim their health and the wonder of their bodies, in all of their abundance.

MAKEUP

At all ages, women are terrorized by the billion dollar cosmetic industry. From birth, women are bombarded with billboards, magazines, and television messages that claim looking young and beautiful and therefore their very being depends upon covering or painting their faces with a particular brand of foundation, blush, lipstick, eye liner, or mascara. The cosmetic hawkers never mention those layers of "makeup" clog the pores and dry the skin. The sales machine keeps the well hidden secret that women's faces are beautiful in and of themselves.

Once, in a therapeutic exercise, I was forced to wear no makeup for a week. I had to take off the mask and look at my face. I will never forget that experience. I looked in the mirror at my naked eyes and saw their sadness and pain from all the messages I had given that face. I had told my face, "You are plain; you are ugly; I have to cover you." That week began the long, slow process of my learning to love the naked face that stares back at me in the mirror.

Another reason for makeup occurred to me when on a work day I saw my friend, Julie, in her legal garb. Her face was painted to do battle for her female client in the divorce court. I saw her the following Saturday, away from the courtroom, with a washed vulnerable face. I realized how difficult it must be for her to have a soft heart, yet do battle for the rights of women and children. In her lawyer's stance, she reminded me of warriors of old, painting their faces to frighten their enemy. Maybe, they painted them to hide their fear?

Some days, I have to do battle, but painting my face is of no value for my enemies are within. My enemies are my fears, my doubts, and my false thoughts, and only God can give me the courage to win that battle.

HAIR

Besides hiding their faces, women have hidden their hair under the cosmetic industry's color of the month. For years, I monthly dumped noxious bottles of chemicals on my head. Then, I sat for the required time, with nose dripping and eyes burning. Again and again, I tried to make me acceptable to myself with something from a bottle.

Several years ago, I revealed my natural hair color, which by then included many strands of silver. Then nine Thanksgivings ago, I was in emotional pain and, with infinite logic, I decided I would feel better if I dumped a bottle of dye on my head and proceeded to do so. Such logic resembles hitting one's thumb with a hammer to forget one's headache.

Now, my hair is restored to its natural state and, since that Thanksgiving, I have not found it necessary to dump another bottle of chemicals on my head. Now, I enjoy my silver hair and, with each new year, I watch as nature adds more of this lovely color.

Fashion has not only dictated the color of women's hair but its length and shape. Hair styles have varied from long and elegant to disheveled, chopped, and mutilated. At times, women's hair has resembled the aftermath of a lawnmower. With such destruction reaped on the feminine head, one wonders if the fashion gods from their Olympic mount were angered by or jealous of the natural beauty of a woman's hair.

I once complimented my mid-fifties friend, Beverly, on her elegant and beautifully styled mid-shoulder length hair. She thanked me and went on to say her sister and work colleagues had told her that for "her age and profession" short hair would be more suitable.

Beverly and I discussed the norms that prevailed in the seventies. In that decade, we had entered the ranks of the professional work force and had abandoned long hair and more feminine dress and took to androgenous dressing, because any connotation of the feminine would be construed as weak and unacceptable in our male-dominated professions. Being feminine and professionally successful were considered mutually exclusive. Now in our fifties and professionally successful, Beverly and I have emphatically reclaimed our feminine selves. We no longer allow ourselves to be masculinized to be considered strong. My friend and I have come to know that when we are grounded in our feminine selves we are most powerful.

Plastic Surgery

Like the cosmetic and fashion industries, plastic surgery is claiming a market share of the "beauty industry" and cutting a wide swath over women's faces and bodies. I have seen movie and television celebrities, after a number of plastic surgeries, look like macabre silicon caricatures of their former selves. Plastic surgery includes face lifts, tummy tucks, liposuction, peelings, scrapings, injections, breast implants, and all the ways we change ourselves because, in and of ourselves, we do not feel lovable.

A few years ago, I saw a dear, long-time friend who had, previously unknown to me, undergone extensive plastic surgery. I was deeply saddened. She was stretched, pulled, peeled, tucked, and barely recognizable. Her face was like a mask. I kept wanting to ask, "Is my friend behind there anywhere?"

I loved her real face, the one with the twinkling eyes that could make the most wonderful expressions, the one that had cried, loved, and laughed. She looked as though plastic had erased her character.

I mourned her real face that was lost to the surgeon's cutting and snipping. I didn't even get to tell that delightful face goodbye.

Beauty and Sensuality

As she approached fifty, I heard a friend bewail her perceived loss of youth and beauty. As she talked, I realized she associated her beauty and sensual self as a function of a dress size or an age.

Webster's definition of sensuality is "voluptuousness," and beauty is defined as, "The quality...that gives pleasure to the senses or pleasurably exalts the mind or spirit." How lovely. There are innumerable ways, unrelated to an age or dress size, we as women give pleasure to the senses, mind, and spirit.

European women seem to have a stronger grasp on this concept than we North American women. Several years ago I visited Italy and the Mediterranean and viewed women of every size, age, shape, description, and nationality wearing single and two-piece bathing suits, with an occasional topless bather. They did not hide their bodies. They were there to bathe and luxuriate in the sea. In their bodies, they had no shame.

Later, I visited an American beach and was shocked by the contrast. Only a few women wore swimsuits without coverups. Most women wore big shirts, shorts, or loose dresses, with an occasional glimpse of a bathing suit beneath. They obviously felt very uncomfortable with their bodies. I felt sad for the shame our society has taught women to have for their bodies. Our European sisters have much to teach us.

RECLAIMED POWER

Women must reclaim their power from the billion dollar industries of fashion, cosmetics, and plastic surgery. Women must also reclaim their power from men and change men's views of them, but men's views of women will change only when women change their views of themselves. If women consider themselves beautiful, sensual, sexual beings at any age and size and without excessive makeup, plastic surgery, or hair contortions, they will be. If women consider themselves bright, capable, and strong, they will be. We become what we think.

If women treat themselves with dignity, love, and respect, they will be treated in like kind, for we teach others how to treat us.

If you don't believe those positive attributes about yourself, act as if you believe them. Change your view of yourself, even if you have to act as if you are a beautiful, sensual, sexual, strong, capable, bright woman. One day, you will realize you are those things and, in so doing, you changed the view of the men in your life.

Beauty has little to do with the external. This attribute is related to the beauty of our souls and how we choose to think and feel about ourselves and others. A beautiful soul radiates divine light and love from every cell and fiber of the body it inhabits, and one's inner radiance is a glorious sight to behold.

CHAPTER NINE

Addictions

HOW WE PERCEIVE THE WORLD determines our responses to it. Addictive behaviors are maladaptive coping skills often developed in individuals with skewed and negative world views. Unfortunately, addictive behaviors are pervasive throughout our society and far exceed the arena of alcoholism and drug addiction, but we will begin there.

The Bio-psychosocial Model is helpful to describe the factors that contribute to the formation of alcoholism and drug addiction. This model identifies the biological, sociological, and psychological factors that contribute to the development of these dependencies.

The biological factor denotes our genetic makeup and manifests as a genetic predisposition to the development of alcoholism or drug addiction once the use of these substances is instituted. When many biological family members have alcoholism or drug addiction, individuals must recognize that they may be genetically prone to have problems with these substances and realize that it would be in their best interest to avoid their use. Individuals who value themselves and have a positive world view are often able to avoid repeating the patterns of their alcoholic and drug addicted family members. However, criticism, low self-esteem, and negative world views are frequently common in the family systems inhabited by alcoholics and drug addicts. Therefore, it is often very difficult to assess the true impact of genetic factors.

In addition to negating family systems, other social factors that contribute to the development of alcoholism and drug addiction include society as a whole and our families of origin which model the use of alcohol and drugs as a means of dealing with emotions and life's problems and celebrations.

When reared in negating dysfunctional family systems and through societal and family modeling, individuals psychologically internalize the use of alcohol and drugs as a method of coping with their inner turmoil. With such rearing, the individual's psyche does not develop emotionally healthy coping skills to deal with their thoughts, feelings, and life stressors. With the emotional anesthesia and/or euphoria often produced with the use of alcohol or abused drugs, the individual's mind begins to associate a particular substance with a desired feeling. Those individuals reared in negating family systems usually do not have the skills or tools necessary to self-engender the desired feelings of empowerment, self-confidence, and sense of well-being that the use of alcohol or an abused substance temporarily provides. The psychological dependency on the desired feeling temporarily produced by the use of addictive substances will often occur long before the physical dependency is firmly established.

The Bio-psychosocial Model is helpful in explaining the factors that contribute to the development of alcoholism and drug addiction. This model takes into account genetic programming, the society and family in which an individual is reared, and the feelings and thoughts the individual psychically incorporates as a result of their rearing in an often negating environment conditioned to the use of alcohol and addictive drugs to interface with the realities of life.

Whether individuals are addicted to alcohol or drugs or just use "socially," these substances have a deleterious impact on everyone. All substances of abuse affect our exquisitely balanced and wired nervous systems. When caffeine, nicotine, alcohol, or other addictive substances are taken into our bodies, it is like hitting our nervous systems with a hammer. We certainly wouldn't treat our home or office computers that way, but we persist in abusing our body's computer system and expect it to function calmly, efficiently, and productively.

In addition, the disorders of alcoholism and drug addiction are cunning, baffling, powerful, patient, and very deadly. Even before the development of dependency, there are many drug and alcohol related deaths, such as acute alcohol poisoning, cocaine or amphetamine related heart attacks or strokes, and automobile accidents.

After the dependency on drugs or alcohol is developed, the death rate goes up, and I have seen many deaths due to addictions. Three particularly come to mind.

On three occasions, I court-committed Leonard to alcohol treatment because of his suicidal thoughts while drinking. After treatment, a smiling, sober Leonard would come into my office and thank me for those commitments. But Leonard didn't make it. One night while drunk and crossing a street, he was struck and killed by a car.

Katherine was a beautiful young woman. While she was pregnant, for the safety of her unborn child, I court-committed her to alcohol treatment. The next time I saw Katherine, she was again pregnant and in a women's drug and alcohol treatment center. She came to my office that second time, smiled shyly, and introduced herself. I hadn't recognized her. In her way, Katherine thanked me for her first court-commitment to treatment. Because of her alcoholism and drug addiction, she had lost custody of her three children, and she wanted to keep her unborn child. She had a beautiful baby boy but, because of her emotional wounds and fractures, Katherine was unable to stay clean and sober. When her son was less than a year old, Katherine was found dead in a dumpster.

Mark minimized his alcohol use. Having been to treatment, he knew all the answers. Besides, he drank "just a little." While drunk, Mark crashed his car and died instantly.

I grieved each death, and those deaths burned into my soul the treacherous nature of the diseases of alcoholism and drug addiction. For these addictions are cunning, baffling, powerful, patient, and very lethal.

PHYSICIAN-AIDED ADDICTION

The rising number of addicted individuals is often unwittingly contributed to by physicians. For instance, patients who seek help from their physician for their anxiety or "nerves" are frequently prescribed and become addicted to benzodiazepines, while the source of their underlying anxiety remains untreated.

Benzodiazepines are highly addictive and include such drugs as Xanax, Ativan, Valium, Librium, Tranxene, Dalmane,

Halcion, and Restoril. A short time after ingesting these sub-stances, the body requires greater amounts of the drug to relieve the anxiety or nervousness. Everyone's body develops a toler-ance to these drugs, requiring an ever increasing dose to achieve the desired calming effect. Eventually, these patients become as or more anxious than they were before starting the benzodiaze-pine. What they are then experiencing is the compounded effect of their underlying anxiety and mini-withdrawal from the drug, with the latter occurring daily and throughout the day. The withdrawal symptoms of anxiety agitation and irritability are relieved only briefly when the drug is administered. Tolerance, withdrawal, and the requirement for more of the drug to achieve the desired effect is the essence of addiction.

Patients can be withdrawn from benzodiazepines quickly while hospitalized or slowly on an outpatient basis. Even with a slow taper, the patient will experience withdrawal. Invariably, once they complete withdrawal, they become calmer, cope, and feel better. Concurrently, the patient's therapeutic tasks are to achieve insight, develop coping skills, and institute life changes to treat their underlying psychosocial stressors that cause their anxiety. These personal changes will often obviate an individu-al's need for non-addictive anti-anxiety medications.

Like benzodiazepine addiction, narcotic addiction is often related to prescriptions issued by physicians in the treatment of pain. Pain is often initiated or exacerbated by internalized emotional stress. To withdraw from and treat a patient who is addicted to narcotics is similar to the process used in benzodi-azepine addiction.

TWELVE-STEP PROGRAMS

Addicts and alcoholics can best cognitively restructure and develop emotional insight and healthy coping skills through the twelve-step spiritually-based programs of Alcoholics Anonymous and Narcotics Anonymous. These programs consist of men and women who share their experience, strength, and hope with each other so they can solve their common problem of alcoholism or drug addiction. The members of these programs share how they have recovered from a seemingly hopeless condition of mind and body, and they state that their primary purpose is to stay sober and clean and to help others to achieve sobriety or abstinence.

The only requirement for membership in these twelve-step programs is a desire to stop drinking or using. You do not even have to admit that you are an alcoholic or addict. You just need the desire to stay sober or abstinent.

Alcoholics Anonymous and Narcotics Anonymous have revolutionized the treatment of alcoholism and drug addiction. Many alcohol and drug treatment centers are now available, and the best centers use a twelve-step model and transition their clients into twelve-step programs to ensure the addict and alcoholic's long-term recovery.

The twelve-step programs are spiritual programs based on admitting personal powerlessness and developing a relationship with a Higher Power to achieve and maintain sobriety or abstinence. The first step toward personal transformation of any kind is to admit personal powerlessness. Most people struggle against their human condition and powerlessness. We humans often behave like tyrannical petty gods or potentates and wear our-selves and those around us out in our struggle to control every aspect of our lives. The fortunate learn they are powerless over people, places, things, and situations and the only person they can change is themselves and, to do that, they need God's help.

The human revolt against the concept of personal powerless-ness is derived, I suspect, from fear, possibly fear of being lost in the morass of the unknown. In believing in a Higher Power or God of one's understanding, individuals receive a beacon in life's storms and the knowledge that God will provide the safe harbor for the floundering vessel of their spirits. So, quit strug-gling. Let go. Surrender. Acknowledge your powerlessness over people, places, and things and allow God's beacon to guide you to safe mooring.

The second step in twelve-step programs is about coming to believe that a Power greater than you are can restore you to san-ity. In this context, insanity is said to be, "Doing the same thing over and over, expecting different results." I know this is not the psychiatric definition, but this statement rings true.

Individuals often repeatedly enact dysfunctional behaviors, including addictions, hoping that this time the behavior will yield the desired results, only to tumble once more to the bot-tom of the emotional scrap heap.

Sometimes individuals get so stuck in their dysfunctional be-haviors that only a power greater than themselves can extricate them from their emotional quagmire. As they begin to rely on a Higher Power, these individuals are restored to sanity, come to believe in that Power, and place more of their lives in that Power's care.

The crux of the restoration to sanity is to rely on a power greater than oneself to help one choose healthy thoughts, behaviors, and attitudes. That ought to be sanity in anybody's book.

For their recovery, addicts and alcoholics are recommended to do the following to maintain their abstinence and sobriety:

+ They regularly attend Alcoholics Anonymous or Narcotics Anonymous meetings. Frequently, they attend ninety meetings in their first ninety days of sobriety or abstinence, and three to five meetings a week thereafter.

+ They get a sponsor. A sponsor is someone who lives the twelve-step program and has been sober or clean for at least a year. This person acts as a guide to help the alcoholic or addict learn to live by the principles of the twelve steps of Alcoholics Anonymous or Narcotics Anonymous.

+ They daily pray only for the knowledge of God's will for them and the power to carry out that knowledge.

+ They meditate daily. Meditation is some form of listening to God, which may include reading, quiet times, chanting, walking, or any method to help them quiet their minds and go to their centers.

+ They do not drink or use, no matter what. In these programs there is a saying: "No matter what, you do not drink or use. Even if your behind falls off, you pick it up, put it in a wheelbarrow, and take it to a meeting."

Alcoholics Anonymous and Narcotics Anonymous are free. To have a desire to stop drinking or using is the only requirement for entrance into meetings and to become a member of these blessed fellowships and, if you do not like what these fellowships offer, the members say you can go to the next bar or crack house and get a "refund on your misery."

PROFESSIONAL HELP

Besides the twelve-step programs, alcoholics and addicts often need professional help. After alcoholics and addicts have been sober and clean for a period of time, they may become severely depressed and suicidal. They usually relapse, get professional help, or die.

With continued sobriety and abstinence, alcoholics and addicts may experience the surfacing of feelings and memories related to sexual, emotional, or physical trauma or other unresolved childhood issues. The twelve-step recovery programs are superb, but professional help many often be necessary for some individuals to achieve full recovery.

I have seen individuals recovering from alcoholism or drug addictions refuse to get professional counseling or take medication. They maintain all of their answers can be found in the twelve-step literature and meetings. This is not true. These individuals may eventually relapse or commit suicide. I remember a particularly gruesome death of a woman who had been sober for thirteen years. She set fire to herself.

Some alcoholics and addicts may also have other disorders, such as Major Depression, Bipolar Disorder, Post-Traumatic Stress Disorder, or Adult Attention-Deficit Disorder. Without professional help, these individuals may relapse repeatedly or die.

PSYCHIATRY

As a psychiatrist, I have worked with recovering alcoholics and addicts for more than twenty years. I initially trained and practiced in pathology but, after concluding that I was dealing with the wrong end of the life cycle and much of dis-ease was due to our internalized emotions and the abuse we perpetrate on our bodies, I retrained in psychiatry.

Another reason I became a psychiatrist is that I wanted to be part of the solution. I had often seen psychiatrists treat alcoholics and addicts for Major Depression, Bipolar Disorder, Schizophrenia, or Anxiety Disorder, with their alcoholism and addiction minimized or ignored and left untreated. Likewise, I had witnessed individuals with alcohol or drink-induced mania or psychosis misdiagnosed as Bipolar or Schizophrenic, medicated, and not treated for their primary disorder.

Perhaps, as more psychiatrists become knowledgeable about the treatment of alcoholism and drug addiction, fewer addicts and alcoholics will be over-medicated and shuffled off to mental wards while ignoring their primary disease.

NICOTINE AND CAFFEINE ADDICTIONS

In addition to alcoholism and drug addiction, there are a broad range of addictions which are often considered "socially acceptable." For example, nicotine is as addictive as heroin and does nothing good for the body or emotions.

As a pathologist, I have seen nicotine, tobacco, and smoking's effect from one end of the body to the other. The effects range from the cancers of the oral cavity, lungs, kidneys, urethras, and urinary bladder, to vascular disease with heart attacks and strokes.

Then there is the emotional impact of nicotine and smoking. The drug nicotine directly effects the nervous system and causes depression, irritability, agitation, and anxiety. Also, the act of smoking inhales and stuffs feelings.

Nicotine is a powerful and destructive drug and is as addictive as heroin, but this is not portrayed by the young, sexy women and virile men in the advertisements. If the tobacco industry advertised using the faces and bodies of men and women who had smoked for thirty years, the sale of their products would plummet.

In addition to nicotine addiction, there has been an exponential rise in the addiction to caffeine with the advent of the high-powered caffeinated carbonated beverages, café lattes, and espressos. With caffeine intoxication, one experiences anxiety, rambling thoughts and speech, muscle agitation and twitching, increased heart rate, and insomnia. Also, similar symptoms are experienced in the process of caffeine withdrawal.

SEXUAL ADDICTIONS

Sexual addictions are as destructive to an individual's body, mind, and spirit as any addictive substance. Even though married or in long-term relationships, the sex addict will have numerous affairs and/or compulsive-addictive behaviors such as the use of sexual fantasies, pornography, masturbation, "cyber sex," or even more deviant sexual behaviors. As with all addictions, these behaviors provide temporary anesthesia of the addict's underlying feelings.

Many individuals with sexual compulsive-addictive behaviors have issues based in childhood sexual trauma. For some children who were sexually abused, the only pleasure they experienced as a child was that of orgasm, and they may begin compulsive masturbation at a very early age. Without developing healthy coping skills, as these children mature they may experience the compulsion to escape their life's realities through the euphoria of sexual orgasm. In addition, a sexually abused child develops confusion distinguishing between nurturing, love, touch, and sex. As an adult, their child-self may want to be touched, nurtured, and loved, but those needs are translated into sex.

It has been said that the most powerful hypnotic known to humans is the sexual abuse of a child. The abuse imprints deep messages into the child's psyche. In adulthood, these imprints can manifest as compulsive-addictive behaviors such as multiple affairs, masturbation, pornography, voyeurism, fetishes, and pedophilia.

There are twelve-step programs for sexual addicts. In this day of AIDS and continued sexual perpetration of children, sexual addictions should never be scoffed at or minimized. Along with twelve-step programs, abstinence and recovery from a sexual addiction may require professional help.

COMPULSIVE SPENDING

Compulsive spending is another form of addiction. In spite of continued adverse consequences and debt, the compulsive spender will continue to shop and spend. Because of their addiction, compulsive spenders may be forced into bankruptcy or incarcerated for writing bogus checks.

Even though I had sufficient income, I became a compulsive spender. I was reared in relative poverty and dreamed of a big home filled with beautiful furnishings. As a professional woman, I proceeded to fulfill my dreams. On some level, I thought those possessions would bring me happiness, security, and acceptance.

I obtained the large home and filled it with beautiful furnishings and accessories. I was miserable. The objects were lovely to view but gave me no emotional fulfillment, and some of them were so expensive I felt tense being near them. In my healing, I learned that happiness comes from within and my divine connection. I sold the objects. I didn't own them; they had owned me.

Several factors are involved in the addiction of compulsive spending:

+ There is the rush or high that comes from shopping, spending, and possessing the coveted object.
+ There is the thought, although perhaps subconscious, if one has the "perfect" home, clothes, car, or toys, one will feel happy, valued, and secure.
+ The spending numbs and anesthetizes unresolved feelings and issues and prevents their resolution.

Debtor's Anonymous is a twelve-step program for compulsive spenders. I know when I wanted to stop spending compulsively, I first had to admit I had a problem. Then, each time I walked into a store, I began to pray for God's help to buy only what I needed. Eventually, the compulsion was removed. However, even now, I often take out a little extra insurance and pray before entering a furniture store.

WORK ADDICTION

Our society perpetuates and encourages work addiction. The person who works the hardest and longest gets the accolades. God help a person who gets on the treadmill of success and approval.

Work addiction serves several functions:

+ Compulsive overworking often gives the addict approval
  they did not receive in childhood. The work addict continues to attempt to gain approval from surrogate parents, also called bosses and colleagues.

+ Compulsive overworking can generate an adrenaline
  rush derived from stress and hyper-functioning, and the
  addict becomes dependent on that high.

+ In overworking, the addict avoids dealing with emotional issues and stressful life situations.

In compulsive working, addicts deprive themselves of their
basic human needs for love, rest, relaxation, and nurturing.
Work addiction is emotionally and physically depleting, often
leaving addicts burned-out shells of their former selves.

In recovery from work addiction, the addict focuses on getting off the treadmill, restoring balance, and becoming a human
being, rather than a human doing. Often, work addicts must
be taught to give themselves permission to rest, relax, and play.
They also learn to approve of themselves and that they don't
have to perform for love, that love is their birthright.

COMMUNICATION AND INTRUMENTATION ADDICTIONS

Some people are addicted to being wired for sound. Have
you ever been concerned that the cell phone would take root in
their ear? They seem obsessed with the need to be available to
talk to anyone and everyone from any location and at any time.
Have you ever noticed people who, even with message retrieval
systems in place, will stop whatever they are doing to answer the
phone. I was once married to a communication addict. Even in

the height of passion, he would stop to answer the phone. Talk about a letdown.

Communication addiction has now bumped up a notch, with the sophisticated development of cell phones that can e-mail, play games, dance, and sing. I suspect communication addicts have difficulty being alone with and looking into themselves. The fact that so many people want to communicate with them makes them feel important and helps them remain scattered and externally focused.

The communication and instrumentation addiction extends to computers, the Internet, chat rooms, and video games. These addicts may spend many hours a day in these pursuits. These behaviors are just another form of anesthesia of one's feelings and an attempt to avoid dealing with one's reality.

ADDICTION RECOVERY

If an addiction distorts your world perceptions, consider a twelve-step program. These programs form the foundation of recovery from addictions to substances and behaviors. The result of twelve-step programs is a spiritual awakening or a spiritual arousal from sleep.

Do you feel you have been in a long slumber? At times, have you felt stone cold dead inside?

When people work twelve-step programs, their lights come on. Somebody is finally at home inside. Their step quickens. Smiles appear. They see more clearly. They are awakened to themselves and to God.

If for a long time nobody has been home in your house and an addiction has taken residence therein, consider a twelve-step program, and see about awakening your spirit and tuning in to God.

CHAPTER TEN

Trauma and Its Sequelae

AFTER MANY YEARS OF WORKING WITH THOSE ADDICTED to substances and behaviors, I have realized that addictions are only the tip of the iceberg. Often the addict's core issues are emotional, physical, or sexual trauma.

Twelve-step programs are invaluable in assisting alcoholics and addicts to become clean and sober. In addition, these programs help their members to evolve spiritually and develop healthy coping skills.

However, with severe emotional, physical, or sexual trauma, professional help is often necessary for full recovery. In therapy, the individual becomes acquainted with the huge emotional icebergs that have battered and blocked their life and been capped by the addiction to substances or behaviors.

Various techniques are helpful in the treatment of trauma survivors, including experiential regression work, inner-child work, cognitive restructuring, and spiritual grounding. The therapeutic process releases fear, pain, anger, and the secrets. When the bulky mass of emotion bobbing beneath the surface begins to shrink, it can no longer create a shipwreck of one's life.

In my own life, I almost died from my submerged trauma memory. In 1989, at the end of my second year of psychiatry residency, I became severely depressed and planned suicide. On that pivotal day, I looked into my six-year-old son's face and remembered that the greatest trauma one could perpetrate on a child is the suicide of a parent. I knew I had to get help or die.

Within twenty-four hours, I was on a plane bound for a New Mexico inpatient sexual trauma treatment center. As I boarded the plane, I knew I was going to the center of my being, and my life would never again be the same.

Prior to treatment, I had received years of therapy but could retrieve only a part of one trauma memory. In the first week at the treatment center, I had a one-and-a-half-hour flashback. In a regressed state, I screamed, groaned, and cried as I relived the trauma of a satanic cult ritual. I saw blood and dead animals. I saw my father with a bloody knife and heard my mother screaming for him to kill me. Through the flashback, my roommates touched, stroked, and soothed me. Their grounding presence gave me assurance that I might not be insane and could possibly survive the experience.

The evening after the flashback, as I walked across the courtyard, I felt what seemed like a cosmic explosion of my subconscious mind and saw fragments of memory flying out into the starlit New Mexico sky.

During my thirty-five days in treatment, I had many memories, and my prior reality was shattered. I was unsure if I could ever function again. In a compromised state, I returned home. I had another year left in my residency and was determined to finish. With much prayer and every ounce of courage I could muster, I returned to work. I also became active in individual and group therapy. To the depth of my being, I cried and wailed my grief. I screamed my rage until I was hoarse. New memories surfaced to my consciousness, and I captured them on paper before my conscious mind could again suppress them. I prayed and, one day at a time, I walked out of my nightmare.

Over the next three years, my trauma memories became an integral part of my everyday reality. I embraced my wounded inner child and her true reality. To make her life bearable, this little girl had spent hours arranging her dolls perfectly on her bed. Her dolls were perfectly dressed, perfectly in order, and perfectly still. She did not play. She invented the dolls' lives, and their lives became hers. In my healing, I remothered this inner child, and she now knows a child's joy.

Now, as an integrated whole and healthy being, I walk with my blinders off and my feet firmly planted on the earth. I walk in the sunlight and live at peace with my reality. For you who are afraid of your trauma memories, I invite you into the light.

TRAUMA MEMORY

Trauma memories may surface years after physical, sexual, or emotional abuse. The memories may surface in the form of visual, auditory, or sensory flashbacks. Flashbacks may begin as intrusive feelings of fear, panic, or anger. One may feel discomfort or revulsion at a particular smell, taste, sound, or touch. Certain words or phrases may trigger unexpected reactions. Pictures or sounds may surface into one's consciousness. As the trauma's visual memory retrieval progresses, the memory may appear like a slow movie reel exposing one frame at a time, often accompanied by sounds, smells, tastes, or tactile experiences.

In a full-blown flashback, one may go into a regressed state and re-experience the trauma. This regressed state may last thirty to ninety minutes, and rarely more than three to four hours. This is unlike a psychotic episode, which can last days, weeks, or months. Too often with the uninitiated, a regression may be misdiagnosed as psychosis or schizophrenia.

Trauma memory retrieval enables survivors to claim their reality and unload its associated emotional baggage. Certainly, the avoidance of remembering the trauma and experiencing its resultant feelings has contributed to every known human addiction.

In the individual's and society's avoidance of the reality of the despicable crimes humans perpetrate on other humans, there has been a rash of cases toward therapists "implanting" trauma memory. Some of these cases may indeed have merit, but I suspect most of them are just another form of denial that such fiendish trauma occurs. In my experience, trauma memory is exquisite in detail and specific to the time, place, and life of the individual. None of my memories were "planted." They all came directly from the infinitely detailed records of my subconscious mind.

Satanic Abuse

From the emptying of my subconscious storehouse, I know that satanic abuse does exist. Satanic abuse is a ghoulish form of human degradation and torture that happened to me and countless others. I have lived it. I know it. On occasion, it still haunts my deepest darkest dreams.

Satanic abuse consists of:

Altars, hooded cloaked figures, black nights, full moons, chains, cages, coffins, and graves;

Rituals using feces, blood, and urine;

Torture with snakes, spiders, cats, dogs, cattle, and horses;

Sacrifices of animals, adults, and children;

Rapes, sodomy, and every deviant sexual behavior known to man.

Satanic abuse glorifies and worships evil. I have seen my own memories and heard those of countless others. I have seen its victims from many states, cultures, and socioeconomic levels. This is my reality and the reality of countless others. Satanic abuse exists. I have survived it.

In our society, the hidden cults of satanic perpetrators wear many guises. I once had a chilling sensation as an adolescent recounted to me her weekly three-hour participation in a game about vampires at a local game shop. She described how each adolescent was a vampire character that "frenzied" for blood, survived on the blood of innocent victims, and returned to their coffins by day. In her innocence, this adolescent again reminded me how subtle cults and perpetrators are in procuring their victims.

Within the same week, I heard an adult cult trauma survivor describe how, as a child, she was forced to drink blood and eat raw flesh from both animals and humans. She recounted her burial in coffins. In her experience, individuals abused by cults may assume perpetrator roles by the time they reach adolescence.

As the adolescent proclaimed to me the safety of the vampire game run by adolescents in the game shop owned and run by an adult male, my blood ran cold. I was also reminded that pedophiles are often day-care employees, school custodians, Sunday school teachers, priests, deacons, or scout leaders. They may preside over any activity where their prey congregates.

Trauma's Effects

Through my memory retrieval and trauma healing, I discovered much information to aid me in the understanding of my behaviors and the behaviors of others. For instance, I remembered the barn where as a small child I was raped and sodomized. In that barn my parents and cult members performed rituals and killed animals and people.

When I now take a patient's history, my ears prick up when events are asssociated with garages, sheds, barns, or outdoor buildings. I file that information away with an index of suspicion, because I remember in those buildings things happen to children.

From another of my memories, I realized that I was codependent at age three. This realization came when I remembered that one night from my bed I heard my mother crying. My father was hollering, and I knew he was beating her. In hopes that he would stop, I pretended to be thirsty and went to ask for a drink of water. My father dragged me onto the bed. While raping me, he screamed at my mother, "She can do it better than you."

Codependent behaviors include sacrificing one's own needs in the caretaking of others. To many, I give the "Codependent's

Bill of Rights" (*see Chapter 13*) and encourage them to put it on their refrigerator and read daily for a year. I consider dealing with codependency issues essential in the healing process, and I encourage trauma survivors to read codependency literature and attend twelve-step codependency meetings. I do this, because I remember a little girl who one night asked for a drink of water to take care of an adult.

Other experiences that were my teachers include the day I was playing house on the back porch of our home. Unaware of danger, I sang, chattered, and played with my dolls and dishes. My father came from behind and dragged me into his bed. During his attempt to rape me, I struggled. He violently separated my legs and dislocated my right hip. From that time forward, I stopped playing. I became silent and vigilant. It was not safe to play; he might catch me unaware. This event happened in 1950.

In 1989, after treatment and retrieval of this memory, I began to have recurrently more intense right-hip pain. The pain became so excruciating that I was taken to a hospital emergency room, followed by a five-day hospitalization with tests and x-rays. The orthopedist concluded there were degenerative changes of my spine, but I knew that I had experienced a body memory of the rape and right-hip dislocation at age four.

With myself and others, I have repeatedly seen the phenomenon of body memories. At the time of the emotional and physical abuse, the trauma was too painful for the child self to experience, so the memory was stored in the body at a cellular level. Later the memory surfaces as physical pain, and the trauma survivor may be seen repeatedly in doctor's offices and emergency rooms with chronic, undiagnosable pain of the head, neck, back, shoulders, legs, or pelvis.

As each of my memories unfolded, I began to understand the impact of that particular trauma event on my life. For instance, as a small child on a full moonlit night, I was taken from my bed, placed on an altar, and circled by chanting, dark-robed figures. As I processed this memory, I began to realize why I felt so uncomfortable in gatherings of people, and why I went for years without allowing overnight guests in my home. I understood why I was so selective about who I allowed in my home. They had to feel safe.

With my recovery, though my isolation has decreased, I honor my need for privacy and select with care the individuals I allow into my personal space, for I remember a small child taken from her bed at night and placed on an altar. Now, my job is to keep her safe.

From another memory, I understood my obsessive need for order when I recalled that as a child of four or five I was unable to go to sleep at night until I had meticulously smoothed, without a wrinkle, the chenille bedspread that covered me. This was my childlike way of attempting to protect myself and have some sense of control. Of course, my father still came to my bed.

I have now heard many trauma survivors relate their repetitive hand washing, bathing, cleaning, and clothes-changing behaviors to their trauma. With childhood trauma, the child or—in the case of an adult, the child within—develops repetitive, obsessive compulsive behaviors to feel some sense of control over their internal and external environments.

With another memory, I understood part of my difficulty accepting and valuing myself as a woman. As a preteen, I was forced to perform oral sex on my mother and her mother. The experience was so vile to me that I despised my developing woman's body and its shape, hair, and smell. With my anorexia, I stripped my body of its breasts and feminine curves because it bore resemblance to my female perpetrators. It took me years to begin to like, then later love, my womanness, in all my smells and shapes. This was particularly true of my genitals, which on some level, I believed to be a source of shame and ugliness. With this mindset, many sexually traumatized women develop serious pelvic diseases, including cancer.

The origins of other self-destructive behaviors became apparent with a memory of an event that occurred when I was thirteen. I was forced to lay in a field beside an idling tractor. On the dirt, rocks, and hay stubbles, my father anally, then orally, raped me. Inside, I screamed, "Why is he doing this? Can't he see how ugly I am?" Because I knew he valued beautiful women, I had cut my hair to short brown stumps, gained weight, and irritated my adolescent pimples. Out of my child mind's attempt to protect, lay the roots of what later became my full-blown disorder of compulsive overeating and a recurrent pattern of mutilating my hair and skin.

Self-abusive behaviors are very common for trauma survivors. They may include compulsive hair pulling or cutting, weight gain, bulimia, anorexia, skin picking, and even cutting or burning the skin.

Although unhealthy, the abusive behaviors fulfill several functions:

+ The behaviors act out self-hate and punishment. Because of the abuse, the survivor has internalized the belief that something must be wrong with them to deserve such abuse. From this flawed-self view, the survivor continues re-enactment and punishment behaviors.

+ Disfiguring behaviors often serve as a protective mechanism from sexual attention.

+ By the infliction of physical pain, the emotional pain can be refocused and temporarily relieved.

Self-abusive behaviors block healing. For health and wholeness, the survivor must discontinue these behaviors and experience the underlying emotions.

Many of my trauma experiences demonstrate the phenomena of dissociation. For example, when I was sixteen my father came to pick me up from a school function. I wore a white dress, with a fitted waist and full skirt that I had made myself. He drove me to a motel and anally raped me. Afterwards, I washed the blood and feces from my body, knowing in the morning I would not remember. Indeed, the next morning I dressed for school, made straight A's, and continued in my trance, an automaton. I was locked in the silence of my forgotten memories.

This description is the essence of the dissociation and amnesia found in Post-Traumatic Stress Disorder, which is the result of emotional, sexual, or physical trauma.

Today, I no longer dissociate from my feelings, my body, or my reality, because today I remember, and my truth has set me free.

EXPERIENCE YOUR FEELINGS

Trauma survivors often come to me filled with pain and anger. They fear that if they feel these emotions, the pain and anger will destroy them. However, if these feelings are not released and remain trapped within, the survivor becomes emotionally or physically ill.

In therapy, trauma survivors develop healthy ways to release their trapped feelings. I discuss with them the finite nature of their painful emotions. As long as the survivor is not traumatized, the trapped feelings are like a non-replenishing well. Each piece of work they do, each time they cry or express their anger, their internal well of these emotions is siphoned, and the well's level is diminished. Each segment of anger and pain that is released never has to be re-experienced. There may be other pieces of work related to that segment, but that piece is gone. Each time the survivor feels the anger and pain, the level of the well lowers, and those emotions occupy less and less space within. When one realizes their internal pain and anger can be released one portion at a time, their fear of being destroyed by their feelings is diminished.

When the subconscious mind is ready, trauma memory begins to surface to conscious awareness. These memories do not have to be pushed or prodded. They just come. Often the feelings are so frightening, survivors expend much energy, especially in addictive behaviors, to suppress them. I advise survivors to step back and let the feelings roll through. Often the emotions are so powerful, they feel like a freight train is moving through, but I encourage the survivor to surrender to the pain, anger, and grief. Then step aside, and let the emotions roll through like a locomotive moving on down the tracks. After you have raged, cried, moaned, groaned, and wailed to the depth of your being, something wonderful happens. Healing begins. The freight train comes through less often and with less intensity, and peace, love, and joy take its place.

MULTIPLE PERSONALITY DISORDER

I have worked with a number of individuals with Multiple Personality Disorder, now also called Dissociative Identity Disorder. To survive severe trauma, the child-self splits into multiple inner parts of self, or alters, which are discrete packets of trauma memory and function. These inner parts of self may not be aware of the existence or actions of the other parts of self.

The alters often have different likes, dislikes, abilities, functions, and biology. One alter may go to English class and another to math. One alter may be male, another female. One alter responds to a medication, another does not.

In healing, the alters, or parts of self, become co-conscious of each other. The memory walls begin to dissolve, and the memory becomes confluent. Eventually, the splitting and switching between parts of self decreases and an integrated whole emerges.

With severe trauma, one child-self would be destroyed by all the trauma information, so for survival, an ingenious child-self splits the memory into distinct packets with separate identities. As in many of the trauma survivor's adaptive skills, the switching and splitting become very self-destructive in adulthood. Healing from this disorder is long and arduous, but many survivors make the journey.

TRAUMA AND BRAIN CHEMISTRY

Chronic or severe emotional, physical, or sexual trauma changes the brain's neurochemistry. The information is now considerable on the effect of chronic trauma on the brain. The trauma effects neurotransmitters and the axonal and dendritic development of neurons, which means that with chronic trauma the brain develops and functions differently. Combined with the psychodynamic effects, this change in brain function may manifest as depression, anxiety, panic, and obsessive-compulsive behaviors.

A chronically traumatized child, on some level, lives in a state of constant fear, agitation, hypervigilance, and shock. This state changes the brain's neuro-chemical communication. The child is living in a war zone, a childhood Vietnam.

Traumatized children will have difficulty concentrating, attending to tasks, and may experience episodes of dissociation, which result in school difficulties and further humiliation from teachers and peers. Later in life and to cope with their burden of emotional pain, these children may develop one or more compulsive-addictive behaviors.

Chronic trauma affects the psyche and the brain's neurochemistry. Healing requires remembering, feeling, and owning the trauma and, with healing, the brain's neurochemistry is positively altered. Healing may require therapy, twelve-step programs, and medication. But remember, no matter how severe one's trauma, healing is possible.

TRAUMATIZED WOMEN AND ADDICTIONS

The national average of sexually abused women is about thirty-three percent. Over ninety percent of women in alcohol and drug treatment centers have been sexually abused.

As previously discussed, trauma survivors use alcohol and drugs to numb their feelings. For women recovering from alcoholism and drug addiction to heal emotionally and have long-term abstinence and sobriety, they must deal with their issues of shame and trauma.

As a child is traumatized, they often internalize shame from the verbiage heaped upon them by their perpetrator. In addition, their child mind reasons that there must be something inherently wrong with them to deserve such punishment. To compound their shame, an alcoholic or addicted woman is often treated by society as an unfit mother or bad wife and considered sexually promiscuous. With their compounded underlying trauma and social stigmata, women with alcoholism and drug addictions carry enormous burdens of shame. Because of the associated shame women tend to hide their use and seek help less frequently, and this behavior is often aided and abetted by their male partners.

In the recovery of traumatized women addicted to substances, I have observed two recovery sequences:

+ The woman becomes sober and clean, works a recovery program, and in time the trauma issues surface and are treated.
+ The woman is unable to stay sober or clean. When the anesthesia from drugs and alcohol is removed, the trauma pain surfaces, and the woman relapses because she cannot cope with the pain or memories. These women must be treated for their alcoholism, addictions, and trauma concurrently, or they will be unable to stay sober and abstinent.

For women in the recovery process from alcoholism and drug addiction, their issues of shame and sexual trauma must be addressed in their healing process to ensure long-term sobriety and abstinence. I have seen women recovering from alcoholism and drug addiction who did not receive treatment for their trauma. Many of them relapsed, and some died.

To compound these difficulties, alcoholic women experience more severe medical problems over a shorter period of time and by consuming smaller quantities of alcohol than does their male counterpart. Compared to alcoholic men, alcoholic women experience an accelerated progression of osteoporosis, brain damage, cardiovascular disease, and alcoholic liver disease. In addition, women who abuse alcohol have a higher incidence of breast cancer than their abstinent feminine counterparts.[8] In other words, a woman's body is more vulnerable to the toxic effects of alcohol.

TRAUMA'S GIFTS

For their highest good, trauma survivors must look for the positive perspective in their trauma. I now consider my childhood trauma and its healing journey my greatest gifts. These events brought me to my emotional and spiritual knees, and I had to surrender to God's will and care or perish. To heal, I had to travel to the center of my being, where God resides. By surviving the blast furnace of my pain, my spirit was forged into a durable resiliency. By surviving what many consider the unsurvivable, I now know that when I walk with God there is nothing to fear. For I am always safe and protected.

For my spiritual evolution, I know that the degree of pain I experienced with my sexual trauma was required for me to release my ego driven mind and surrender to Divine Consciousness. Only when my ego driven self was beaten into submission could my divine Self emerge. To walk with God, all of my old ideas, ideals, and ways of living had to change. For my healing and spiritual evolution, I had to surrender my will to God's and, by doing so, my life has been immeasurably blessed.

Because of my trauma and its healing, I am the woman I am today, and for that I am immensely grateful. Because of my journey, I believe, adamantly and irrevocably, that no matter what your trauma you can heal, but healing requires that you surrender all of you to the God of your understanding. When our pain threatens to destroy us, we become willing to surrender, as only those facing death can be. From that degree of willingness, our divine Self emerges. To know our divine Self and experience its union with God is a gift beyond measure.

CHAPTER ELEVEN

Eating Disorders

COMPULSIVE OVEREATING, ANOREXIA, AND BULIMIA are addictions similar to alcoholism and drug addiction. The function of all addictions is to anesthetize feelings. Individuals with eating disorders attempt to accomplish this anesthetization by binging, purging, and/or restricting food. In the United States, eating disorders have reached epidemic proportion and are fueled by the dictates of fashion and our society's skewed values regarding the feminine and masculine form. The dilemma is further compounded by our media's bombardment of our consciousness with visual stimuli to tempt the palate and, after the consumption of such taste treats, one is condemned for their caloric intake. To arrest this epidemic, our society must change its approach to food and its perceptions of masculine and feminine attractiveness.

To cope with the emotional distress of my childhood sexual trauma, I developed an eating disorder. My behavior was characterized by periods of anorexia alternating with periods of compulsive overeating. I did not purge. However, I am certain that if purging had served an emotional need, I would have done so.

In my anorexia, I stripped my body of all vestiges of womanness. I had control over my body and its breasts, hips, and thighs. I made them disappear. Then, I looked like the fashion models, therefore I must be valuable and acceptable.

Eventually the day arrived when I could no longer sustain my anorexic level of starvation. I would begin to binge and gain large amounts of weight. On my surgery rotation in medical school, my emotional pain and depravation were so great that I gained fifty pounds in six weeks.

By compulsive overeating, I attempted to obliterate my consciousness with massive quantities of food. With the weight gain, I shrouded my body from sexual attention or predators. With the excess mass, my inner child self felt strong and impenetrable and said, "I am big. You can't hurt me." Being full of self-hate, binging also served as a means to flagellate myself.

The eating disorders of anorexia, bulimia, and compulsive overeating are psychodynamically complex and interconnected. My eating disorder, and that of countless others, had its roots in childhood trauma. However, with God's help and the help of many professionals, I recovered from my eating disorder. If you are so afflicted, I hope my sharing will help you.

BEAUTY'S FORMS

To halt our national epidemic of eating disorders, our society must begin to value, love, and find beauty in people of all shapes and sizes. In doing so, our verbiage must become more positive and life affirming. For example, we beat ourselves with the word "overweight." What in the world does that word mean? Over what, a weight?

In my practice, I see individuals concerned about being "overweight." Their healing involves learning to love themselves exactly as they are. I discourage "dieting" and encourage them to choose healthful foods and exercise out of love for themselves. I ask them to delete self-negating words such as "fat" and "overweight" from their vocabularies.

My female patients and I talk of a woman's body being made to have soft, round, and lush breasts, hips, and thighs. We discuss the beauty of the full body of womanness and of feeling beautiful at any shape or size. We also discuss the social conditioning that formed our Barbie Doll mentality.

In working with women with anorexia, my message is the same. I give them permission to exist and have breasts, thighs, hips, and the roundness of womanness. These women are encouraged to release all restrictive food behaviors and given permission to nourish and love their bodies with healthful foods and behaviors.

For men with eating disorders, I use a similar approach. For the message remains, regardless of gender, that we are each divine and beautiful creations, and we must treat ourselves accordingly.

From social conditioning, many women and men have dieted in attempts to fit their forms into our society's standards of attractiveness. I encourage all my patients to abstain from the use of "diets," because diets don't work. This fact has been reported and proven over and over by me and you. The word "diet" even implies to die.

Certainly, diets have taken many forms, including, to mention only a few, all-protein, all-liquid, all-vegetable, all-fruit, and fasting. There has been the Atkin's Diet, the Pritikin's Diet, the Grapefruit Diet, and the Dieter's Diet. Dieters have counted calories, proteins, fat grams, and carbohydrates. They have counted and counted, looking for that magic number to make them acceptable to themselves.

Dieters have used the scales, tape measures, and body-fat measurements to determine if they were a success. Dieters have also measured their success by the way a mirror reflects their appearance in a swimsuit, pair of jeans, or a particular dress or suit, as if any number or object could determine one's success.

Because of objects and numbers, dieters have called themselves fat, ugly, or gross. Because of their "weight," many people have hated themselves and wanted to die.

Have you ever believed if you called yourself enough names and beat yourself with enough objects, you would lose weight, but instead, you gained more? Did you ever say to yourself, "Oh well, if I am fat, I might as well eat?"

I believe the opposite behavior is much more successful. Get rid of the tight jeans and dresses. With the scales, I recommend you bury them or run over them with a truck. Cutting and burning works nicely for tape measures.

No matter what your size, clothe your body and spirit in garments that look and feel beautiful. Tell your body how much you love it. Tell yourself you are beautiful and your body is glorious and divinely made. Whether you believe the words or not, repeat these affirmations every time a negative self thought enters your mind.

Stop beating your body and spirit. Claim your power from numbers, words, and inanimate objects. Every day, tell yourself how beautiful and wonderful you are, and treat yourself as if you believe it. You might be surprised one day, for our subconscious mind hears and manifests everything we tell ourselves.

RECOVERY TOOLS

Numerous types of support and therapy groups are helpful in recovering from an eating disorder. One very powerful group is Overeaters Anonymous, a twelve-step program modeled after Alcoholics Anonymous. For those in Overeaters Anonymous, their drug of choice is food.

Overeaters Anonymous is a spiritual program. Members develop a relationship with a power greater than themselves to help them do what they cannot do alone. Having the ability to eat in a healthful manner, without compulsion or shame, is only one manifestation of this "Higher Power" in their lives. Overeaters Anonymous is a fellowship of men and women who together share their experience, strength, and hope. Members work twelve steps based on universal spiritual principles. Through deep self-examination, the members come to know their emotional makeup. Then, they work to release the emotional baggage and behaviors that hold them hostage and fuel their addiction. Overeaters Anonymous is not a diet club. It helps its members stop binging, purging, and/or restricting food as an emotional buffer from the world. Overeaters Anonymous helps individuals with eating disorders to relegate food to its true purpose—nourishment.

Overeaters Anonymous uses the term abstinence. Each individual has their own definition of abstinence. Abstinence is the set of guidelines within which each individual desires to eat. Abstinence might include counting calories, following a food plan, or simply eating three moderate meals a day.

Overeaters Anonymous can help the compulsive overeater, the bulimic, and the anorexic. All of these disorders are a continuum of the same emotional process. The anorexic and bulimic share with the compulsive overeater a distorted body image and the dilemma of what, when, how much, and what kind of food to eat or not to eat.

In addition to support groups, there are many excellent books to assist in one's recovery from an eating disorder. Geneen Roth's books have been an excellent teacher for me. Her lessons were simple but changed my life. I received the following in her writings:

Eat when you are hungry.

Stop when you are full.

Eat what sounds good.

Do not count calories, fats, or carbohydrates.

And for me, I added, "Do not weigh and measure myself." In her writings, I read about our body's divine wisdom and was taught to listen to that wisdom. Roth writes that our body knows what it needs to eat and what size it needs to be. What a concept. The billion dollar "weight loss" industry has kept the truth well hidden.

The writings of Geneen Roth are a blessing and a teacher for me. However, my greatest teacher has been my own body in its infinite wisdom and divine connection. Everything I need to know about what I need to eat is revealed to me by my body and its inner knowing. I must only listen. My body, and yours, contains divine wisdom, which we must learn to honor and follow.

BARBIE DOLLS

Barbie Dolls are a woman's greatest nightmare. With their long legs, full breasts, "perfect" hourglass waist, and just-right hips, they are a mythical form of feminine perfection.

Where are the Barbie women? The gyms, aerobics classes, and weight-loss clinics are full of women trying to achieve this illusion. I have seen only a few women who achieved Barbie's form, and that achievement required food restriction, excessive exercise, plastic surgery, and significant emotional dysfunction.

Study the great artists such as Titian, Rubens, Renoir, and Matisse. Their works abound with voluptuous, rounded female forms sitting, standing, reclining, clothed, and unclothed. The women of these artists are luscious and ripe.

Then we come to today's boxes of stiff plastic dolls, with perfect mix-and-match wardrobes and anorexic fashion models plastered throughout the media. Our conditioning is completed by beauty pageants for all ages, including toddlers, teens, Miss, and Mrs. From birth, we are bombarded with distorted images and expectations of womanness.

Stop. No more. Women, be your own Matisse and enjoy yourselves in all your shapes and sizes.

THINKING ERRORS

We often live our lives on erroneous assumptions or thinking errors. This fact was evident as I facilitated a women's group in which one member stated that if she were "thin" she would:

look younger,
have more energy,
be more vivacious,
look more professional,
be more acceptable.

Though depressed, the woman looked young and beautiful and was a highly regarded professional.

As the group explored these statements, they concluded that being vivacious, accepted, and looking more professional had little to do with thinness but more to do with feelings of self-worth and projecting those feelings outward. With the current incidence of anorexia and bulimia, thinness certainly is no indicator of physical or emotional health.

Thinking errors are often encouraged by the media and advertising's attempts to market the current diet product, image, or lifestyle. In life's times of transition and growth, we must examine the assumptions by which we live. We must identify and rectify our errors in thought.

"As Is"

How often have you set conditions on yourself before you would participate in an activity? Did the conditions require you to lose weight, let your hair grow, firm your thighs or abs, or whatever it was that would make you fit into the form of a department store mannequin, replete with shrunken cheeks and a stick waist?

A woman once recounted to me her preparation for a long-awaited date. After spending anxious hours dressing, undressing, and redressing, she finally mentally put on an "As Is" sign, went out, and had a wonderful time.

Shortly thereafter, I was delighted by a wonderful magazine, "Mode," dedicated to real women. The issue contained a two-page advertisement with a reclining couch occupied by a nude Barbie. The doll had full rounded hips, thighs, and belly. The only thing lacking was an "As Is" sign.

◎ ◎ ◎

Recovery is possible from an eating disorder, but recovery requires changing your entire perspective and attitude toward food and your body. Recovery also requires the healing of your emotional wounds and brokenness. A good therapist, a support group, and Geneen Roth's writings can be most helpful. Going within and connecting with your divine wisdom is essential.

CHAPTER TWELVE

The Inner Child

THE INNER CHILD IS THE PART OF SELF that enacts obsessive compulsive behaviors such as compulsive spending, cleaning, lying, eating, working, and the compulsive use of alcohol, drugs, and sex. These behaviors result from the need to control, repress, or annihilate unwanted thoughts, feelings, or memories. These behaviors are the inner child's attempt to relieve or anesthetize their reality.

The inner child part of self functions as the repository of unresolved pain, fear, anger, and forgotten memories. The inner child part of self is pure subconscious mind. Everyone has one or more inner children. Because of the extent of my trauma, I had several. However, when an inner child was present the remaining parts of myself were co-conscious, unlike the amnesia that exists between parts of self in Multiple Personality Disorder.

Oftentimes, in our biologic adulthood, the inner child part of ourselves slides forward and functions in our daily lives, under the guise of an adult, and engages in obsessive compulsive behaviors to anesthetize feelings and repress memories of unresolved mental, physical, or sexual abuse. For example, due to unresolved anger, the child self may have anger outbursts or throw tantrums related to seemingly minor incidents that occur at home or in the workplace. Guised as an adult, the operant inner child may make impulsive, irrational decisions. Through memory retrieval, one travels to one's center and releases the long festering pains, fears, and angers. As these feelings are cleansed from one's psyche storehouse, the childhood wounds heal, and the healthy nurturing adult becomes the predominant part of self that operates in the workplace and in personal relationships. With healing, the inner children become a confluent integrated whole, and the child's natural joy begins to bubble forth.

When we are reared in dysfunctional families, we often internalize a punitive parent which continues to neglect and abuse our inner child self. With inner child work, we learn to re-parent ourselves. The punitive parent is the part of self that calls you "stupid, fat, ugly, and a failure." I encourage patients to banish their punitive parent part of self to a mental closet and work on developing a healthy affirming adult self that gives their inner child the love, attention, acceptance, and praise they didn't receive in their biologic youth. In this process, we become our own best parent and our own best friend.

In re-parenting, one replaces the negative messages of childhood with positive messages such as "I love myself; I am beautiful; I am intelligent." Re-parenting is a process of learning to treat all parts of oneself with dignity, love, and respect.

INNER CHILD DEVELOPING

To re-parent, one must learn their inner child's thoughts, needs, feelings, likes, and dislikes. This information retrieval can be assisted with right- and left-hand dialoguing. If right-handed, the adult self writes with the right hand and the child self answers through the left, or the reverse if the adult is left-handed. If the developing healthy adult self listens, the inner child will reveal its truth.

When I was in trauma treatment, I began right- and left-hand dialoguing. As my inner children disclosed their existence, they began to reveal to my adult self bits and pieces of trauma memory. The first response of my adult mind was often to disbelieve the information, but I knew that I must be open to the possibility that what the children were writing was true. As the inner children began to trust my adult self to tend them and accept their truth, the memories came in visual flashes. Often, they would begin as a single frame or picture, which over time unfolded like an exquisitely detailed movie reel. The visual memory was sometimes accompanied by the associated feelings, but often these feelings were delayed and released in a collective manner at a later date.

At times, in releasing my pain, I knew I needed to cry, but I didn't know why. I learned to "cry into it." I learned that if I allowed the tears and feelings to surface that bits and pieces of memory would begin to play through my inner vision like news clips, and I became aware that I was experiencing collective grieving from numerous trauma events.

Likewise, when random anger began to surface, I would beat my bed with a tennis racket. As the anger energy rolled forth from me and onto the bed, a myriad of incidents attached to that anger would come to mind.

If you are plagued with obsessive-compulsive behaviors, get out your pen and paper and begin to dialogue with your inner child. Ask, with your dominant hand, what the child likes, feels, thinks, and needs? Let the child write back with your non-dominant hand. As the child reveals to you, the healthy adult self, its feelings, thoughts, and longings, be sensitive, nurturing, and responsive.

I was tested on my responsiveness when I returned home from trauma treatment. I felt like a raw wound, as if my skin had been ripped off. During that period, I happened to see a large, beautiful, blonde doll in a toy store window that resembled the one that had burned in the fire that destroyed my childhood home when I was six. My inner children screamed to have it. The doll cost $250.00. My adult self initially resisted but knew she had to purchase the doll for her wounded inner children. We all went home with the doll that day. To release feelings and to retrieve trauma memory, the doll along with several teddy bears were my lone companions through many regressions.

FOOD AND THE INNER CHILD

As I began to work with my inner children and their food issues, I discovered the interplay between the restrictive, punitive parent and the deprived and rebellious inner children, and this interplay set me up for a binge.

In 1992, after a long period of rigid food rules and restriction, I began to binge. My healthy adult self knew she had to change. Through the help of Geneen Roth's writings, I began to release my and society's rigid rules regarding diet and a woman's body shape. Using Roth's guidelines, I began to eat when I was hungry, eat exactly what I wanted, and stop when I was full, and I did not count calories or measure me or my food. With no threat of deprivation or restriction of their favorite foods, the inner children could pick and choose what sounded and felt good. I realized, when the punitive parent part of self restricted or deleted sweets, for example, from my food intake, internal pressure began to build. When the inner children finally broke through my punitive adult self's rigid wall of control, they gorged themselves on their treasured foods, because they knew it would be a long time before they would get to eat them again. When the children were free to pick and choose what they wanted to eat, the binging was no longer necessary, because the children knew they could eat whatever they wanted when they were hungry.

If you watch a young child eat, you know they are usually very picky eaters and only want to eat what tastes good to them and, unless trained to overeat, they refuse food when they are full. Unless already conditioned to compulsively overeat by the adults in their lives, the only time you usually see an older child gorge themselves is when they are eating something they know they will not be able to eat again for some time.

When I allowed my inner children to eat when they were hungry, to stop when they were full, and to eat exactly what they wanted, my binging ceased. Without the rigidity and restrictions of the punitive parent, the inner children had no need to binge. Also, as my inner children tested and explored their freedom, they became very selective about what they would eat.

Over time, I also discovered that if the child self thought they wanted chocolate or sweets for a meal and ate it, they didn't feel good afterwards, which resulted in their making that choice less often or not at all. To avoid feeling bad, the children began to select and eat pleasurable but more healthful foods and, with these choices, they discovered they felt better. Eventually there developed a healthy internal balance between the body's intuitive wisdom and what it needed for nourishment and the needs of the inner children and the healthy adult self. In fact, no parts of myself like many of my former binge foods. If I eat a dessert, I want the best quality of my favorite sweet and not something purchased at a convenience store.

During my trauma healing, if my inner children wanted food and hunger was not the issue, I dialogued with them, asking them how they felt. I often found they were feeling neglected, tired, or stressed. The children were then offered enjoyable healthy alternatives to meet their true needs. Their needs could usually be simply met by a walk, bicycle ride, movie, hot bath, or just time alone with my adult self to rest, relax, and be nurtured. During my healing, I discovered it takes very little to nurture these bruised and wounded inner children. With my eating disorder, I learned out of extreme emotional deprivation, pain, and anger, my inner children were the part of me that binged. They wanted something, anything, to make them feel better.

As you become acquainted with your inner child or children, you will discover their needs are simple and that they are often easily pleased and highly distractible. In being reared in a dysfunctional family, the child self developed unhealthy thoughts and behaviors to deal with life stressors. In healing, the adult self identifies the child's triggers and responses and begins to offer the child healthier behavior choices.

Often, with an obsession, the child self is feeling stressed and neglected. Rather than acting out obsessive-compulsive behaviors, increase the adult and child self's repertoire of healthy choices. When dealing with an obsession, listen to the inner child and identify the distress. In lieu of a compulsive behavior, divert the child's attention to healthy choices, and then, go play.

SPONTANEOUS COMMUNICATION

During my trauma healing, I frequently used right- and left-hand dialoguing. Eventually, spontaneous internal conversations began to occur between the healthy adult and the child parts of myself.

As these inner parts of self began to freely internally communicate, they negotiated their needs and the sequence and manner in which these needs would be met. There were many times in that first year following my inpatient trauma treatment that I would receive frames of a flashback while at work. Rather than immediately going into a regressed state and retrieving the remainder of the memory, my adult self would internally negotiate with the inner child that was the repository of the memory and promise to allow the flashback to surface as soon as work was completed and we were safely home. With such negotiations, the child self was honored and tended and the adult self could continue to work and function. With such promises, immediately upon arriving home, I would collect my stuffed animals and dolls around me on my bed and allow myself to go into a regressed state. Often in a fetal position, the inner child associated with the event would come forward and reveal the trauma. As all parts of me began to trust this process, the memory was accompanied by the feelings, and I often cried and wailed to the depth of my being. After carrying these memories and their associated pain for decades, I found relief and subsequent joy came with as little as thirty minutes of regression work.

During this period, I sometimes had fragments of a memory that needed birthing, but I could not access it on my own. I would relate these fragments to my therapist. Then, she would say these pieces of memory back to me, repeating them over and over in a soft, melodic voice. With the comfort of her presence, I could then go into the memory and see and feel the trauma event. As each memory came to my awareness and its associated feelings released, I realized that I was siphoning off my internal well of pain.

With memory retrieval through regression work, right- and left-hand dialoguing, grief, and anger work, childhood wounds will heal. As the child self reveals its fear, hurt, anger, and secrets and is tended by the nurturing adult self, the child part of self is re-parented and a loving harmony develops between these parts of self. In this process, the child self develops trust in the nurturing parent part of self to love, protect, and care for them.

Once the secrets are told, the repressed feelings released, and the child self re-parented with loving kindness, much of the driving force behind the obsessive-compulsive behaviors is relieved. This does not preclude the need for twelve-step programs, but nurturing of the child self does help heal the underlying emotional wounds.

In my recovery, my healthy adult self nurtured and tended my inner children and honored their memories. My healing required me, in my totality, to travel to the center of my being and remember my childhood and experience and release its associated emotions. In this process, I owned my childhood reality, and my inner children integrated into a confluent whole.

In healing, the healthy adult self re-parents the wounded and deprived inner child parts of self and gives the child or children the kindness, love, and nurturing that they did not receive in their biologic youth. If you have a wounded inner child or children, remember, it is never too late to have a happy childhood. You can begin now by re-parenting yourself.

CHAPTER THIRTEEN

Relationships

HOW WE RELATE TO PEOPLE, PLACES, OR THINGS in our lives defines our relationships, but these relationships are incapable of being our source of happiness, self-worth, or security. These feelings can only be derived from our relationships with our inner Self and God, which means we need to change our perspective from an outward to inward focus. However, before we are able to direct our gaze inward, we often must traverse a circuitous healing journey.

CODEPENDENT AND DYSFUNCTIONAL RELATIONSHIPS

Individuals reared in dysfunctional family systems, which may include family members with alcoholism and/or drug addiction, may become codependent. Codependency is often defined as the chronic dependency upon people, places, or things outside oneself to feel happy, secure, and valuable. Codependent relationships are pervasive in our society. For personal and societal health, we must change our perceptions of and our relationships with our external environment.

A codependent individual often depends upon a person, be they a parent, boss, spouse, or child, to give them feelings of self-worth, approval, and security.

Codependency upon things can manifest as the need for certain clothes, houses, cars, or jewelry to provide feelings of self-worth and validation.

Codependency on a place can manifest as the need to live in a certain neighborhood, city, state, or country to feel safe, accepted, or worthwhile.

In their quest for validation and approval, highly successful codependent adults often retain an umbilical cord ready to plug into the next available person, job, or situation for nourishment. These individuals persist in demanding their needs be filled by people or things outside of themselves. However, until they begin to nurture, nourish, and love themselves exactly as they are, they will never be happy.

Often as children, codependents were not told that they were wonderful, beautiful, unique beings. In their rearing, they internalized that they were defective and incomplete in and of themselves but, if they had the right things or people in their lives, then they would be acceptable and possibly loved.

Along similar lines, relationship addiction is described as an individual's constant need or compulsion to be in a relationship with a "significant other." Often, when they are in such a relationship, they lose their identity and become absorbed in being who and what they perceive their partner desires them to be. The relationship addict often becomes consumed with meeting the needs of their partner, to the exclusion or detriment of their own needs.

In her writing, Robin Norwood seems to have at least partially explained this phenomenon of relationship addiction. She writes of women who had emotionally unavailable, or even abusive, fathers who continue to seek, in their male partners, men similar to their fathers in an attmept to receive the love, nurturing, and approval they did not receive as children. The converse is also seen with men reared by emotionally unavailable mothers and the women they partner.

I also find that relationship addiction has its roots in the fear of being alone: the fear that alone one cannot care for oneself or that one is not whole in and of themselves.

In addition, when individuals are reared in and the survivors of dysfunctional families, which may or may not include a family member with alcoholism or drug addiction, they often recreate an environment which feels familiar to them, so they often surround themselves with toxic people in the form of employers, friends, spouses, and even their children. Toxic people spew out so much anger, criticism, and negativity that being in their presence is like sitting under a factory smoke stack belching out environmental pollutants. For survivors of dysfunctional families, toxic people treat them in the manner in which as children they were conditioned to be treated and, if the people that surround the survivor do not naturally treat them in the manner in which they have internalized that they deserve, on some level the survivor teaches them.

Growing up as emotional punching bags, survivors of dysfunctional and/or alcoholic families were not taught that it is their God-given right to be treated with dignity, love, and respect. As bruised and battered adults, these survivors often reach a time in their lives when they can no longer tolerate the mental and sometimes physical abuse of others. In their healing, they learn to treat themselves with love and dignity, and to demand the same treatment from others.

When being precipitated upon by an emotionally toxic individual, healing survivors learn to state their boundaries and then remove themselves from the offending individual. With the onset of verbal abuse from another, the survivor might say something like, "I will not be spoken to in this manner. When we are both calm and you can speak to me in a respectful manner, we can resume this conversation." After setting this boundary, the survivor may remove themselves from the presence of the abusive individual and, sometimes in the case of aggressive spouses or partners, this removal may consist of staying overnight in a hotel room. As survivors treat themselves with dignity, love, and respect and maintain their boundaries of being treated in like kind by others, they retrain the people in their lives. For we teach others how to treat us, and students always learn by the teacher's example.

Sometimes, the individuals with whom the survivors have surrounded themselves resist the teacher's example. In this case, the survivors must own that they are not a victim but a volunteer and that they have chosen their emotional environment. With this realization, they are empowered to make another choice. They can continue to choose to remain in the company of angry, critical, negating people as they spew forth their emotional poisons, or they can choose to remove themselves from the hazardous fallout zone, be it a marriage, job, family function, educational or social setting.

The survivor of a dysfunctional family may decide, for various reasons, to remain in the company of the negating and critical person. In such circumstances, the survivor must develop skills in self-care and internally detaching themselves from the individual's demeaning words and behaviors. The survivor must realize that the words and actions of an abusive individual are not about the survivor but about the individual producing them. For a support group and to improve one's relationship skills, Alanon and Codependency literature and meetings can be invaluable.

Alanon and Codependent's Anonymous are twelve-step programs that have an excellent body of literature on healing the codependent and individuals in relationships with alcoholics and addicts. These twelve-step programs focus on the individual developing an affirming, approving, and loving internal relationship with themselves. To this end, the individual begins to value and approve of themselves exactly as they are and ceases giving their power to something or someone outside of themselves. Also, in their healing, they develop a relationship with a Higher Power on which they can rely to meet their needs.

Since early childhood, I had codependently taken care of and tried to control people, places, and things to help me feel safe and loved. In 1986, I was an Assistant Professor of Pathology at the University of Oklahoma Medical Center. I was in crisis and burn-out. Needing help, I entered a thirty-day codependency treatment program in Arizona. The experience was life changing. I began to honor myself, my feelings, and my inner knowing. Before leaving treatment, I knew my work in pathology was over. Within the year, I began my second residency in psychiatry.

In the codependency treatment center, I received a copy of the "Codependent's Bill of Rights." The fact that I had rights was a revelation to me. After returning home, I posted my "Rights" on the refrigerator and read them daily for a year. In that time, I internalized the following rights and made them my own:

+ I have a right to express my feelings.
+ I have a right to express my thoughts.
+ I have a right to say no.
+ I have a right to agree or disagree with another.
+ I have a right to change my mind.
+ I have a right to make mistakes.
+ I have a right to say, "I don't know."
+ I have a right to be treated as a valuable human being.
+ I have a right to have my needs met.
+ I have a right to not be responsible for the feelings or behaviors of others.
+ I have a right to my choices.
+ I have a right to make my decisions.
+ I have a right to play.
+ I have a right to joy and happiness.

What freedom. I had a right to say what I felt and thought. I had a right to say no or disagree. I had a right to change my mind, make a mistake, and not know the answer. Amazing. I certainly had not been taught my rights in my home of origin or in medical school.

Before codependency treatment, I had spent my entire life feeling as if I was a kid outside the candy store with my nose pressed against the window, looking at the other kids on the inside enjoying the good stuff. The "Codependent's Bill of Rights" helped me open the candy store door, go inside, and like Forrest Gump, buy my own box of chocolates.

In addition to codependency and Alanon literature and meetings, there is the twelve-step program of Adult Children of Alcoholics. After being reared in alcoholic homes, adult children of alcoholics often experience a constellation of similar thoughts and behaviors. These thoughts and behaviors are also often manifested by individuals reared in dysfunctional family systems, without the presence of alcoholic family members.

Woititz and others have described the following characteristics of Adult Children of Alcoholics:
+ They have to guess at what is normal.
+ They have difficulty following projects through to completion.
+ They judge themselves without mercy.
+ They have difficulty having fun.
+ They take themselves very seriously.
+ They have difficulty with intimate relationships.
+ They feel different from other people.
+ They constantly seek approval and affirmation.
+ They are either super responsible or irresponsible.
+ They avoid conflict or aggravate it, but rarely deal with it.
+ They fear rejection and abandonment, yet they reject others.
+ They fear failure, but have difficulty handling success.
+ They fear criticism and judgment, yet criticize others.

Like the twelve-step programs of Alanon and Codependent's Anonymous, Adult Children of Alcoholics is a spiritual program modeled on the program of Alcoholics Anonymous. The literature and meetings help the survivors of dysfunctional or alcoholic families to identify their individual dysfunctional thoughts and behaviors and to develop healthier behaviors and skills. Of course, many of the characteristics of adult children of alcoholics overlap with those of a codependent and relationship addict.

Whether the twelve-step program be that of Alanon, Adult Children of Alcoholics, or Codependent's Anonymous, the survivor's healing journey includes discovering that their nourishment comes from within and through their divine connection. Each individual must learn to love and nourish themselves and bask in all of their sublime humanness. Then, so resplendently nourished, they can release the last vestiges of their umbilical cords.

LETTING GO

"Letting Go" is a concept found in most of the twelve-step program literature. I once heard a woman declare to her spouse, "Consider yourself turned over." The woman's declaration turned her spouse over to God, because she finally realized she could not fix, control, or change him, so she let him go into God's keeping.

How many times have you connived and manipulated your spouse or partner into doing or being what you thought they ought to do or be? How did it work? In my experience, not too well.

Have you ever been in a relationship and struggled, pushed, and pulled to make it work? Have you kept saying, "If I just do this," whatever this was, "things will be better?"

How many times, after letting go, relinquishing your control, and turning your spouse, partner, or loved one over to God have things worked out better than you could have imagined?

We individuals reared in dysfunctional families are taught to believe if we just do everything well enough and long enough, we will be nurtured and loved. But the harder we try, the further behind we get. When we finally stop struggling, let go of our need for control, and say, "Thy will, not mine, be done," we can bathe in God's abundant love.

Before codependency recovery, I always worked hard for second best. In my healing, I learned my God wants the best for me, but I am required to let go of control and accept God's gifts, which may sometimes come in the form of pain.

Letting go of the adults in our lives also means letting them take responsibility for their behaviors and choices and experience the consequences of their actions.

Frequently, well-meaning parents continue to extricate adult children from financial, emotional, and legal scrapes. These parents "enable" their children in dysfunctional behaviors by preventing them from experiencing the consequences of their actions. These parents also give their children the underlying message, "You are not competent to take care of yourself; therefore, I must do it for you."

The twelve-step programs speak of "tough love" and "detachment," which also means "letting go." These concepts help give relief to individuals who are distraught after attempting, often unsuccessfully, to remedy the results of choices of another adult. If you ever feel yourself being wrestled to the emotional mat in trying to caretake another adult, find a twelve-step program and let go. Let the dependent adult in your life experience their own maturation.

As one evolves and develops an awakened and perceptive mind, every relationship, be it codependent or otherwise, can be a teacher of what we do or do not want to be, do, say, or become.

We might consider releasing or distancing ourselves from relationships that drain, deplete, or negate us and do not serve our highest good. Relationships to maintain and cultivate are those that nurture, enhance, and amplify our emotional and spiritual evolution.

How we relate to or connect with the people, places, and things in our lives defines our relationships, but these relationships can never be our source of happiness, self-worth, or self-love. These feelings are derived only from our most important relationships, the ones we have with ourselves and God.

LOVING THE SELF

Love is the answer to all of life's dilemmas. Learning to love ourselves, in all our humanness, will transform our lives.

As a child, I did not feel lovable, but I believed if I could be good enough and do everything well enough, my family would be happy, and the bad things would stop happening. Out of my family's dysfunction was born my perfectionism, work addiction, anorexia, and my desire to control everything and everyone in my life. These were my inner child's attempts to meet my family's standards. Eventually, after performing to exhaustion, I realized that I would never receive my family's approval. Over time and much healing, I came to know the validation I sought could be found only within me. Thus began my long journey in learning to love myself.

In learning to love and be kind to myself, I was forced to release my unobtainable standards of perfection, with which I regularly flagellated myself when I fell short of their benchmark. The phrase, "Good is good enough, " helped me release my perfectionism.

This saying came to me in my second year of medical school, in which my class consisted of more then one hundred honor students. In our studies, we were thrown together in a pressure tank and forced to compete with each other for recognition and feelings of self-worth. In our drive for perfection, none of us could accept being less than number one.

In this pressure tank, my module mate, Lynn, saved me. I always wondered before exams why Lynn could joke, laugh, smile, and generally enjoy himself? One day, Lynn held forth on his philosophy of test taking. Lynn had wisely realized that there was no point in fighting with the pack for the top positions, so he had settled back to learn the information without being test score driven. In Lynn's thinking, as long as he was learning the material a relaxed C was good enough and, from Lynn's philosophy, I coined the phrase, "Good is good enough." This truth hung over my desk where I spent countless hours studying and, each time I became overwhelmed by that day's upcoming exam, I looked up, read my slogan, and gained some modicum of relief.

Other lessons followed in my third year of medical school. In this year, we trained on clinical rotations in patient wards such as surgery, internal medicine, and pediatrics. We made daily rounds and traveled in a hierarchy, wearing white coats and stethoscopes. There would be the chief resident, intern, fourth-year medical student, and then us lowly third-year students. These rounds were often giant "Gotcha" sessions. We students would be bullied, battered, and humiliated for our fledgling store of medical knowledge, and the more I was battered, the more fearful I became, and the less I could remember. Of course, the person who recited the answers, like a windup toy, got the "Jock Doc" award. I finally concluded that medical school was the last "male virility rite."

As a medical student, I knew I was getting the worst assignment on the ward when I was told the assignment would be "a learning experience," which translates as "manure rolls downhill." The medical school teaching method was one of bullying, battering, and humiliating, the opposite of how I, and most people, best learn. When my turn came in academia and I taught medical students, I advised them to be kind to and take care of themselves, because they were just enduring male rutting season.

After graduation from medical school came four years of pathology internship and residency. I was finally getting paid. There had been four years of college, four years of medical school, and then another four years of residency before I could practice independently in my chosen profession. I believe medical training is the ultimate form of delayed gratification. There is always one more training program, certificate, or exam before one arrives and is designated as "good enough."

Throughout my training and in my quest for self approval and love, I had to reclaim my power from the almighty number. In our society, we often harshly judge and limit ourselves because of lines on a piece of paper.

Have you ever felt good or bad about yourself because of a number you weighed or a clothing size you wore? Trash the scales and cut out the labels.

Have you ever felt you were not smart because of an IQ score or test grade? Never allow grades or the questionable validity of an IQ score the power to limit your thinking or your possibilities. Follow your dreams.

Have you ever predicated your success by the number of dollars you have earned? The number in a bank ledger will never be an indicator of your worth. We are not commodities whose value can be determined by a price tag. When you feel good about whatever you are doing, you are a success.

Have your ever felt old when reminded of your age? I once told a man to change his age from 75 to 57, and he would feel better and stop limiting himself. He did. It worked.

Give yourself a break. Life and love are not measured by a number, and neither are you. Reclaim your power from those lines on a piece of paper and love yourself exactly as you are. Remember, you are God's creation.

Likewise, we give negative words incredible power in our lives. We use such words as "stupid, fat, or ugly" like baseball bats. We often don't have a clue how to be kind to ourselves.

Kindness goes a long way with ourselves and others. Have you ever seen someone blossom before your eyes when you compliment them on the way they look or the job they did? Our spirits also blossom when we compliment ourselves. When we are kind to ourselves and others, it is like tending a rare and beautiful plant which can only thrive and grow in a safe and supportive environment.

Not only do we need to release the unkind words we call ourselves, we need to release negative or limiting judgments that others impose upon us. Once, I stopped writing because I gave power to one person's unkind words.

Similarly, have you ever given a presentation, taught a class, or performed in an activity in which ninety-nine percent of the audience thought you were wonderful and you were criticized by one percent? To whom did you listen? On whose comments did you dwell? Unfortunately in our society's quest for the illusion of perfection, we often listen to the one percent.

With my writing, I had given all my power to the words of another and did not honor or remain true to myself. If the criticism has merit, I must ignore the harshness and learn from the truth, but sometimes those unkind words have nothing to do with my, or your, performance. Sometimes, they are more of a reflection of the inner-world of the person speaking.

When I get derailed by listening to those critical few, I must return to my center and check out my truth. If my writing feels right to me, then it is. I have then reclaimed my power and am listening to the voice of my inner truth. Please listen to yours.

ASSETS

In learning to love and honor ourselves, we may realize that we are our only asset and begin to treat ourselves in that manner. I have often mused on the fact that we are sometimes required to list our assets for banks and credit agencies, and we proceed to list cars, homes, savings, stocks, and bonds. I believe we should list our names at the top of the column.

When I really think about it, I am the only asset I really have. From my mind, body, and soul issue all that is important in my life, and the same is true for each of you. The way I figure it, comfortable shoes and clothes, healthful food, vitamins, toothpaste, dental floss, and every single item I use to care for me ought to be tax deductible as a business expense. Out of my and your healthy beings issue our work and the income on which we are taxed.

Likewise, if we treated ourselves as well as we treat our prized possessions, we would all feel better. Have you ever spent the day cleaning and vacuuming your home for evening guests, only to eat whatever was on hand and wearily throw yourself together before the doorbell rang?

Have you ever carefully placed your computer in the correct temperature and humidity, covering it to protect each precious megabyte, only to place yourself in whatever physical or emotional conditions that blew your way?

Have you ever polished, waxed, and tuned your car to perfection while smoking a cigarette, drinking a beer, or eating junk food?

Stop. You have your assets backwards. You have forgotten, neglected, and abused your only real asset.

As our primary asset, we often need to take action for our self-care or healing or to just take care of business, and we rebel, procrastinate, or drag our feet. We do not want to do what needs to be done. So what. Do it anyway.

As adults, we often let our inner children drive the bus that is us into the ditch, because our inner children do not want to eat their vegetables, stop smoking, exercise, or do whatever is needed to responsibly tend ourselves.

Often as adults, we have to take the child out of the driver's seat, mentally sit it beside us, stroke its head, tell it what a wonderful child it is, but take control of the bus. So if you hear yourself say, "I need to, but I don't want to!" say "So what," and do it anyway. Then, go exercise. Eat healthful foods. Relax. Get adequate rest. Tend your main asset, YOU.

The Audience

In your quest for approval, did you ever feel like a puppet on a stage? Did you perform, sing, and dance so the audience, whomever they were, would approve of you, so then you could approve of you?

So often we continue to play out the scenarios of our childhood, seeking the approval we did not receive as children. In adulthood, we seek validation from bosses, spouses, friends, and individuals in positions of power. We stay on that stage, performing to exhaustion. Inside we are screaming, "Somebody, anybody, approve of me."

Self-approval can only be found within. No matter how much others approve of us, their approval will never be enough. Only when we begin to love and accept ourselves exactly as we are, in all of our wonderful humanness, will we ever have enough of that commodity called approval.

In learning to love and accept ourselves exactly as we are, we shift our perspective from the external to the internal. Then, we can get down from the stage, relax, and take a seat in the audience. Approving and loving ourselves is all we really ever wanted.

PART THREE

More About Healing

CHAPTER FOURTEEN

Our Bodies

OUR BODIES, MINDS, AND SPIRITS are an interconnected whole. However, practitioners of Western medicine often treat them as if they are three unrelated units. Illness or "dis-ease" is a spiritual wake-up call to examine the totality of one's being. After practicing in Western medicine for over thirty years, I know that proper diagnosis and medications may be helpful, but true healing requires physicians and their patients to approach themselves and others as harmonic or, in many cases, disharmonic whole of body, mind, and spirit.

As a practicing pathologist, I experienced this body-mind-spirit split while attending Tumor Boards. The Tumor Board members, often garbed in white coats, included surgeons, oncologists, radiation therapists, and pathologists. The board met to discuss problematic cancers occupying spaces in patients' bodies. With each presentation, a clinical summary of the patient was given, which included the patient's age, gender, previous surgeries, radiological findings, and the histology of the tumor. (*The tumor's histology is its microscopic cellular appearance, which determines the type of tumor and gives some idea of how it might behave.*) After the presentation, board members discussed the patient's general medical condition and the various treatment protocols available for that patient's type of cancer. After some deliberation, the members of the board recommended what additional surgeries, radiation, and chemotherapy they considered best for each patient.

For eleven years, on a weekly basis, I attended Tumor Boards. In that time, I never heard a discussion of the patient's emotional status or spiritual belief system or how these factors might assist in determining the patient's response to therapy. Unfortunately, the Tumor Board was treating the tumor, not the patient, and often the patient was treated as if they were the tumor.

Likewise, during these Tumor Boards, I did not hear a discussion of how dealing with cancer and death on a daily basis emotionally impacted the board members. Sometimes, with unusual and rare tumors, there was almost a macabre fascination. I suspect intellectualization and detachment were the ways the members coped with the fact that a horrifying and often lethal tumor occupied a space in the body of a child, adolescent, young adult, or someone their own age. The board modeled, "Cerebralize, don't feel." If they treated the patient as another case in the protocol columns, a statistic, perhaps they did not feel so impotent with their paltry tools of beams of protons and electrons, knives, and chemicals.

Certainly, all members of the board were dedicated physicians and well-meaning in their attempts to eradicate each patient's cancer. Sadly for their patients, emotional and spiritual healing tools were not among these physicians' armamentarium and, in their minds, a discussion of using such tools in the patient's healing would have been considered weak and unprofessional.

When one realizes that the body, mind, and spirit are a unified whole, one can regard any life-threatening illness as a call to examine one's choices, thoughts, and belief system.

Regarding the body's health or lack thereof, the enlightened masters have long held that the mind and its thoughts control the body. Now, cell biologists are beginning to elucidate the biological mechanism of this ancient truth. In his book and video series, Bruce Lipton, a Ph.D. cell biologist, succinctly describes how our beliefs, thoughts, and perceptions determine our health at a cellular level. He describes each person's body as a "macromolecular ballet" composed of a community of cells numbering in the trillions. He relates that each cell has a nervous system, digestive system, and musculoskeletal system and is finely sensitive in perception and feeling.

Lipton describes that for years conventional scientific thought has held that the genetic DNA of the nucleus of each cell functions as the cell's brain. However, in recent history, cell biologists have shown that in the absence of a nucleus, a cell can live, grow, move, and communicate normally for over two months. Therefore, the nucleus cannot be the brain of the cell.

Lipton emphasizes that the cell's nuclear DNA has no intelligence and is not the source of life but is like the reproductive gonad of the cell. Each cell's nuclear DNA functions to provide the blueprint for the order in which to assemble the twenty-one essential amino acid building blocks to form the approximately seventy thousand proteins necessary for the construction, maintenance, and health of each cell of our body.

Lipton illustrates that cell biologists have determined that the brain of the cell is its outer covering or cell membrane, which responds to the human mind's perception of its environment. The cell membrane, like the brain and the skin, is derived from the ectoderm of the developing embryo. Citing ground-breaking research, Lipton illustrates that the cell membrane of each cell of the human body responds to signals created by the human mind's beliefs and perceptions. When the cell membrane receives signals based on the mind's perceptions and beliefs, the cell membrane effects a behavioral change in movement, configuration, and/or production of cellular proteins. So, the behavior of a cell is not programmed in the nucleus, but is a function of the cell membrane's response to signals generated by the thoughts of each individual's mind. Based upon receipt of a signal or thought perception, the cell membrane relays a message to activate the genes necessary to produce proteins to maintain the cell under the human brain's perception of its environment. The activated gene's DNA is a blueprint for the amino acid sequences required to produce the perceived required protein. Genes cannot self activate so, for example, a "cancer gene" cannot turn itself on. The gene's activation is secondary to the sentient cell membrane's response to the human mind's thoughts and perceptions of its environmental stimuli.

The information received by each cell membrane of the trillion member community of cells that form each human body is not determined by the environmental stimuli, but by how each person's mind perceives the stimuli. How we perceive or what we believe our environment to be is the signal received by each cell membrane of our body. Cell biologists also have demonstrated that through our belief system and our perception of our internal and external environments, our body's cell membranes can select and even rewrite genetic coding to produce the proteins necessary to respond to our perceptions of our world. So our perceptions control the behavior of each cell in our body, the expression of our cell's genes, and can even change the genetic coding within each cell.

Lipton's narrative is astonishing in its impact and validates what the healing community has long held to be true: The human mind is very powerful and what we choose to think and how we choose to perceive our world determines our health. Now through the work of cell biologists, the mechanism of action has been elucidated in how our perceptions of our external and internal world determine the behavior of every cell in our body in every moment of every day of our life. This information is the basis of Lipton's disclosure that ninety-five percent of cancer is related to our perception of our environment and not to heredity.

Lipton discloses that negative thoughts which result in anger, fear, and stress put the body in a "fight or flight" mode and shut down the body's immune system and the body's potential for growth and health. With a fearful, angry life view, our body's cells shut down and go into an energy conservation— survival mode. Every day, billions of our body's cells wear out and need to be replaced. When we choose critical, frightening thoughts which result in similar feelings and actions, the body's healthy process of growth, repair, and replacement of these worn out cells or parts of cells is suppressed, and our bodies deteriorate.

Lipton further relates that loving and kind thoughts and actions and looking for the positive affirming aspect in all of life's circumstances promotes growth, repair, and replacement of cells and enhances our cellular genetic makeup. In essence, our bodies are continually recreating themselves based upon our belief system. So, if we perceive our environment as nurturing and supportive and ourselves as healthy, strong, vibrant beings through all the years of our life, that is the message our body's cells receive and manifest.

What we think and therefore how we feel and act sends signals to each cell of our body. Depending on what we choose to think, our bodies receive the life-enhancing signals generated by love and peace or the toxic and destructive signals generated by anger, fear, and self-hate. When we pollute our bodies with the latter emotions, the cell membranes of every cell of our body translate these signals into susceptibility to illnesses at a cellular level. These illnesses include infections, autoimmune disorders, and cancer. In health, our body's immune surveillance cells identify and attack foreign substances or cells. They do this to safeguard the perimeter. They are the body's security guards or Doberman pinschers.

Our toxic or negative thoughts create toxic feelings that can destroy us emotionally, spiritually, and finally physically. In autoimmune disorders, the cells of the body's immune system attack and sometimes destroy other cells of the body. In these disorders, it is possible that when one dumps toxic emotions, especially self-hate, into one's body, the body's cells respond by a change in their configuration and become distorted and appear foreign to the surveillance cells. The surveillance cells do not recognize the distorted cells as self, so they attack and destroy them.

Furthermore, in the body's normal process of cell division and maintenance, aberrant and even malignant cells are occasionally formed. In healthy bodies, the immune surveillance cells identify and destroy these aberrant cells. When we are stressed, angry, worried, or afraid, our body's security guards malfunction, and aberrant and malignant cells are allowed to grow and reproduce.

As visualized under the microscope, cancer cells often have large aberrant forms, with irregular cell membranes and bizarre shapes of nuclei. Cancer cells no longer function in the healthy community of cells, but go off helter-skelter and proliferate and destroy the cells around them and eventually themselves. Under the microscope, cancer cells could even be said to look emotionally disturbed or psychotic.

In addition to Lipton's work on the macromolecular plane is the research of Dr. Masaru Emoto on the simple molecule of water, which comprises seventy percent of the adult human body. In his book *The Hidden Messages in Water*, Dr. Emoto provides evidence of the impact of our words and thoughts on the crystalline structure of water. With water exposed to words or phrases, either written or spoken, such as "Love," "Gratitude," "Thank you," or "You're beautiful," the water forms beautiful crystals. The same is the case if the water is exposed to the music of Beethoven, Mozart, or Chopin, whereas under the same conditions, if the water is exposed to the words "You fool," "Hate, " "War," or heavy metal music, the crystals are malformed and fragmented.

Emoto's and Lipton's work emphasizes our body's exquisite sensitivity to every aspect of our internal and external environment. How careless we are as we pollute ourselves with self- or world-negating words or thoughts which generate similar actions and feelings. In addition, we often mindlessly place our bodies and souls in places filled with chaos, anger, and negative information blasting from radios, computers, and televisions. In our lack of awareness, we unwittingly destroy our bodies and, when our bodies succumb to illness, we run to a "doctor" to cure us with such crude tools as chemicals, knives, and beams of energy. In our fear-based search for health, we often ignore the most precise healers, our thoughts and our relationship with God.

THE EXCEPTIONAL PATIENT

To counteract these destructive thoughts and emotions, authors such as Louise Hay, Ron Roth, Bernie Siegel, and Gerald Jampolsky write of the healing power of love. They advocate releasing thoughts that generate fear, anger, and resentments. They write of learning to love ourselves and others as a means to cure any dis-ease, including cancer. These authors also give examples of the healing power of prayer and the importance of one's belief in God or a Higher Source.

In treating cancer and other life threatening illnesses, Drs. Jampolsky and Siegel talk of the "exceptional patient." When diagnosed with cancer or other serious illnesses, the exceptional patient takes charge of their life and healing and often explores multiple means of healing besides traditional Western medicine. They explore healthy nutrition and cleansing their bodies of toxic emotions and substances. They visualize their bodies as healthy and free of disease and focus on loving thoughts, laughter, prayer, and reliance on God.

The nonexceptional patient is dependent, needy, and wants someone else to fix them. They go from doctor to doctor and clinic to clinic hoping to find the magic cure, rarely looking within themselves and determining why they are getting their cosmic wake-up call. The nonexceptional patient is often oblivious to the workings of their inner world or unwilling to choose to exert the effort to change their thoughts and attitudes and to place their trust in God. These patients think they are hopeless and weak, and what they think they become.

Love, laughter, positive thoughts, and God can heal us, but only we can choose to be an exceptional patient. Even more importantly, only we can choose to be an exceptional person.

CANCER

As a practicing pathologist, I graphically observed the effect of thoughts and actions on every aspect of the human body. While performing autopsies, the destructive effects of nicotine, alcohol, and diet were obvious. Also, the death of many patients with "cancer" often revealed the nature of their thoughts and life.

I distinctly remember an autopsy I performed on a woman with a huge cancer load, meaning metastasis throughout her body. With the extent of her cancer, she lived years longer and more productively than anyone would have expected. Her life defied logic. I was told she was very cheerful and active, and until a few days before her death, she took care of a man who was wheelchair bound.

Then I recall other autopsies of patients with "cancer," who had died with negligible tumor load. Often, I was unsure why they died. Perhaps they believed they were going to die, and their bodies complied.

From these autopsies, I realized our relationship with God and our attitude toward other people, life, and ourselves have much to do with the outcome of that thing called "cancer," or for that matter, any illness.

Human beings often give excessive power to the word "cancer." With the utterance of that word, I have repeatedly seen individuals paralyzed by fear, resigning themselves to death.

I once saw a strong, vigorous man, after hearing that he had an elevated PSA (*Prostate Specific Antigen*), immediately begin accepting his pending lack of a sexual life and subsequent death. Later, his prostate biopsy was benign. With his thoughts, he had polluted several days of his life.

Once, a healthy appearing elderly gentleman, with the lowered head of resignation, shared with me that his doctor told him he had cancer and had one to two years to live. The gentleman died on schedule.

On another occasion, a gardener was told by his physician that he had pancreatic cancer and had six months to live. The gardener thanked his physician for the information and refused chemotherapy or radiation treatment. Instead, he continued to do the work he loved—tending flowers. Every few years, the kindly gentleman would visit his doctor. The man was an enigma to his physician. God only smiled at the physician's folly.

If you think your life as you know it is over, it probably is. If you think you are going to die in one to two years, you probably will. Every cell of our body listens and responds to our thoughts.

Too often, an individual with a diagnosis of "cancer" is regarded by themselves or others as the "cancer," and is ignored or shunned. Instead, if they are viewed as a divine living being with a tumor occupying a space within their bodies, the balance of power is shifted from the word "cancer" back to the individual.

Too often, when a doctor tells a patient they have a designated time to live, it becomes a self-fulfilling prophecy. But the exceptional patient will delete the information. On some level, they make their own decisions about living and dying and, whatever time they have on the planet, they are truly alive.

CHAPTER FIFTEEN

Our Minds

AS WE HAVE DISCUSSED, OUR MINDS ARE VERY POWERFUL. What we choose to think results in our feelings, actions, and health. Let us look more closely at the emotions of anger, fear, and pain, which are generated by negative self and world views.

ANGER

The emotion of anger results from negating thoughts, conscious or subconscious, toward oneself, others, or life circumstances. When we harbor anger, our behaviors vary, but they are never loving and healing.

One form of anger includes sarcasm masked as jokes, kidding, or teasing that leaves you bleeding on the floor, wondering what happened? Webster defines sarcasm as, "To tear flesh...a sharp and often satirical or ironic utterance designed to cut or give pain." When someone seems to be joking with or teasing you and you are not laughing, check yourself for blood or missing body parts. Chances are you have just been the victim of anger shrouded by "humorous" sarcasm.

Actions of an angry person include criticism, judgment, and fault-finding. With internalized anger, they often have nothing good to say about anyone or anything, and with their biting and unkind words, they foul their and others' emotional environments.

In its most brutal forms, unresolved anger generates rage, hate, violence, suicide, murder, and wars. To cease such world mayhem, it is each individual's responsibility to learn appropriate and healthy means of anger release and resolution.

Often resolution of frustrations, irritability, and anger can be accomplished by re-framing our thoughts regarding the subject in question. For example, if your internal dialogue says "Dave always irritates me," you have given Dave the power to control your feelings. But you may be surprised to find your anger dispelled by changing your inner dialogue to "Bless Dave's heart. He is doing the best he can."

In many instances, individuals need constructive release for their anger before they can begin to restructure their thoughts. Frequently, people are terrified to feel their anger, because they fear it will destroy them or someone else. So, they hold it in, smile, and say they are "fine," and their bodies become emotional time-bombs, or their anger comes out sideways dumping on an unsuspecting passerby.

Anger is a normal human emotion. Only when anger goes unexpressed, or is expressed inappropriately, does it harm oneself or others. Constructive forms of anger release include talking, journaling, writing letters, and hitting pillows, beds, or stuffed chairs with hands, tennis rackets, or plastic bats. Anger energy can also move out of the body by vigorous exercise such as walking, jogging, and biking.

Therapeutic anger release must be expressed in a safe place and not directed toward anyone. In addition to movement, I en-

courage externalizing anger through sound production, especially screaming and profanity. Yes, in appropriately directed anger
work, I encourage profanity. We often stuff thoughts and feelings that bother us because they do not sound pretty. However,
you can be certain these thoughts and their resultant emotions
do not feel pretty, so why should they sound pretty? In a safe
setting, for oneself and others, verbalizing helps externalize long
held rage and resentments.

If anger goes unexpressed, we hold it in knotted stomachs,
tight chests and throats, spastic necks and backs, and clenched
jaws. With talking, writing, movement, and sound production,
we can loosen our energy blocks and empty our emotional
sewer line. When we learn to flush out anger in therapeutic
ways, we stop dumping raw sewage into ourselves and onto
others.

With long held anger, it is cleansing to experience and release the anger in a constructive focused manner such as I
have described. However, with daily life events, we choose
the thoughts that result in the feelings of anger. For example,
have you ever gotten angry when cut off in traffic or by someone barging ahead in the grocery line? Have you ever chosen to
make an obscene gesture or rude comment toward those individuals? I doubt if you felt very good when you chose to pollute
your mind with negative thoughts that resulted in angry feelings
and rude behaviors. When people barged in front of me while I
was on foot or in a car, I began to realize that some people just
need to go first and, when I yielded the right-of-way to them, I
felt better. As they hurried on, I also realized that when I said
something like, "God bless them, or God love them," the angry

bullets ricocheting in my head were replaced by kind thoughts and tranquil feelings.

With the perception of greater offenses toward one's personhood, releasing the anger or festering resentment may require daily prayer for the good and well-being of the individual. These prayers are accompanied by sending them God's blessings and love whenever the perceived offending party comes to mind. When I pray for someone that I think has wronged me, I surround them with God's light and love. When we replace anger producing thoughts with prayers and blessings, we change how we feel and act. Also, what we send out returns to us manyfold. So, if you send out God's light, love, and blessings, they return to you multiplied.

Fear

If you look beneath an individual's anger, you usually find fear, usually fear that they will not be thought well of, fear of losing what they have or not getting what they want, or fear for their own safety or the safety of their loved ones. It is believed by many that there are only two primary emotions, love and fear; however, I would add the third emotion of pain.

The emotion of love is the essence of God and our divine inner Self, as opposed to our ego self that operates on fear. As shown by Bruce Lipton's work, if we choose to live in ego and fear, we choose declining health of body and mind. Whereas, if we choose to live with loving thoughts and hearts, our total being responds in kind.

In his book *Love Is Letting Go of Fear*, Dr. Gerald Jampolsky states that health and wholeness can be viewed as inner peace and that healing occurs when one releases fear. Jampolsky further holds that when we trust the Divine Source and release fear, our spirits bask in God's healing light and love.[9]

The feelings of stress, anxiety, worry, and panic are just fear dressed up in other names. Unfortunately, these feelings are the stock and trade of the "Worrier." These individuals come replete with hand-wringing, nervous stomachs, and back aches. They seem to thrive on news of upcoming bad weather, murders, natural disasters, and wars. Worry, anxiety, and stress are based on fear, especially fear of loss of control. Worriers live in the illusion that they have control.

The best treatment for fear garbed under any name is God. When one surrenders all of their fears to God or a Higher Power of their understanding and seeks to improve their conscious contact with God through prayer and meditation, peace replaces fear.

I much prefer to trust an infinite God rather than my finite mind to find solutions for my life's dilemmas. Over the years, as I gave my life and will to God's care, I have been awed by God's brilliance and timing. With God's help, I find that good can evolve from even the most tragic of circumstances. After observing such transformations, I realized that good and God are everywhere and in everyone. With such knowledge, my fears ease, and I now trust God's infinite wisdom and love in every aspect of my life.

So, if you find yourself in panic and gripped on life's steering wheel, try praying for God's help and wisdom. Then let go, and trust God to take care of you. Prayer works, and so does God.

When we let go and let God take control of our lives, amazing events begin to occur. Such an incidence occurred in my first semester of medical school. Shortly after I received my acceptance letter, it dawned on me that I had to take human anatomy. I was gripped with fear. Then I decided I could handle about anything, except dissecting the human head.

When anatomy class rolled around, we were told that we would be dissecting the human cadaver in teams and, on my team, I was told that I would dissect the head and neck.

My team's cadaver was an elderly African-American woman and, as I worked, something special happened. Each evening as I prepared for dissection and removed the moist cloth from her head, I began to notice the regal shape of her face and neck. She reminded me of the bust of the Egyptian queen, Nefertiti. As I dissected the muscles of her face, I was awed by her grandeur, and we communed together. This experience taught me once again that if I face my fears and walk through a seemingly negative situation, God has something special waiting for me on the other side.

Procrastination is another form of fear. Often, when we look at a large project as a whole, such as learning a skill, writing a paper, cleaning the house, or completing a work assignment, we become overwhelmed and fear that we are not up to the task. So, we procrastinate beginning the project or get stuck in the middle of it. However, if we divide the project into a number of smaller, prioritized, sequential tasks, the fear dissipates, and the feat is often accomplished with relative ease.

Pride is another form of fear, often the fear of looking foolish, incompetent, or not being thought well of. In fear masked as pride, we present a facade to others, so they won't see how inadequate or insecure we really feel. With prideful stances, we often alienate others and isolate ourselves. However, when we allow others to really know us, we usually find that they have fears, insecurities, and concerns similar to our own.

Besides pride, fear that we are inadequate or of little importance parades itself as jealousy and envy and manifests itself in anger, criticism, and gossip.

Fear cloaked as prejudice is a close cousin to pride. Often, the basis of prejudice is fear that we are not "good enough," whatever that means. So, to feel secure in and of ourselves, we prejudicially claim to be superior to others based on our race, education, or financial status. Prejudice is also based on being threatened by and fearful of the unknown, be it a religion, culture, or issues of safety. So, out of prejudicial fear, we enslave and disenfranchise others and deny them their basic human needs and God-given rights.

The fear of not possessing what we want, which far outstrips our needs, generates selfishness and greed. We in the United States consume more than our share of the world's goods, while others in our country and abroad live in hunger and poverty. Certainly, if we, the members of the planet, collectively protect the environment and work to live in harmony and peace and treat each other with kindness, compassion, and love, the planet would supply all of its children's needs.

Rampant fear, masquerading as pride, prejudice, distrust, insecurity, selfishness, greed, envy, and anger, results in illness, poverty, hunger, death, wars, and mass genocide.

Fear has been described as an "evil and corroding thread" that is woven throughout the fabric of our existence. Certainly, the antidote for fear is God. When we believe in a God of love that wants only the best for us, we can fearlessly traverse the path that lies before us. I know my God can take manure and grow roses. How about yours.

PAIN

Negative mind sets are propagated by our society and dysfunctional families of origin. From these negating environments, many people carry heavy burdens of emotional pain. These walking wounded go to work, support their families, and pay their taxes. They are your neighbors, your friends, your workers, and you.

Over time, some of these wounded souls carry their pain directly to God and find solace and healing.

Others attempt to find relief through compulsive-addictive behaviors, including the use of alcohol and drugs. The fortunate among them find emotional and spiritual healing through their religious beliefs or twelve-step programs.

Others in pain seek wise counsel, which might include mental health professionals. In their healing, they learn to feel and release their pain, and they too hopefully develop a strong reliance upon the God of their understanding. Through rigorous labor, these wounded eventually birth themselves, and we in the helping professions act as their midwives. The birthing of these wounded spirits into health is a beautiful sight to behold. Their lights come on. Their smiles appear. Their bodies straighten. But as in any birth, God's handprint is unmistakable.

Besides being emotional and spiritual midwives, therapists and psychiatrists are often emotional surgeons. From unresolved emotional or physical trauma and their associated thought patterns, individuals often carry internal wounds that fester and will not heal until they are pierced and cleansed. The individual often protects the wounded site and does not allow anyone to touch it or them. The road to emotional health is not around but through the pain. After years of carrying their infected walled-off wounds, emotional surgery entails them moving into their pain and crying to the depth of their being. As in the lancing and draining of any abscess, after the wound is washed clean by tears, it heals.

To heal these wounds, life tends to present us with painful circumstances. At such a time in my life, my thoughts and behaviors were very rigid, and I felt that life threw me against a wall and that I shattered into a thousand pieces. I now know that shattering was necessary, and I am grateful for my breakage and the way God brought me back together with new vision, movement, breath, and life.

At times, individuals come to me in crisis, with huge wellings up of emotion. In terror, they fear if they feel their emotions, they will "fall apart." I smile, encourage them to let the pieces fall, and assure them the Master Potter is realigning them into a more creative and beautiful whole.

Frequently in my trauma healing, my emotional pain became so great that I had the intense compulsion to commit suicide. Instead, I prayed, held on, and cried and wailed to the depth of my being. After such times, I began to experience an unfamiliar feeling, joy. As I continued to release my pain, joy became a frequent visitor.

With unresolved pain, I have too often witnessed its results. One day, on arriving at a rural clinic, I was handed a phone

message from a mother telling me three weeks earlier, her fif-
teen-year-old son had ended his life. I was stunned. What
prompted that young life to end? Though from a highly dysfunctional family, he had not seemed as depressed or troubled
as many youth I have known. When I last saw him there had
been no indication that he was suicidal.

How does one ferret out the labyrinth of the mind and
prevent such needless death? In those momentary thoughts
of suicide, the decision lies between the thoughts, their owner, and their relationship with God. To my patients, I repeatedly say, "No matter what do not hurt yourself. Don't quit
before your miracle." I and others can light the path of hope
and healing, but only the individual can make the decision to
live.

After healing from my trauma, I fervently believe that no
matter what your pain, you can heal. So, when patients come
to me in pain, I encourage them to move into and through their
pain. I also strongly encourage them to pray to the God of their
understanding for help but, if they are afraid of their angry, pun-
ishing God, I tell them to fire the sucker and get a new one that
is all loving, all caring, and wants only the best for them. For I
know the Universal God of peace, love, and kindness will cradle
them in their hours of need.

Moving through and releasing one's pain requires shedding
tears. I often hear people say they do not cry because they have
to be strong for mom, dad, sister, brother, child, or spouse. I believe just the opposite. Crying is a sign of strength. To cry and
reveal our vulnerable frail selves takes courage. When we cry, we
give the people around us permission to release their tears and

be human. Crying is the greatest form of strength. So, be strong for the ones you love, cry.

In 1986, a therapist asked me, "What are you running from?" Immediately to my mind came a wall of water towering above me, ready to collapse on my head. I knew the water was my tears and, if I cried, I was afraid I would drown. What followed that question was thirty days of inpatient codependency treatment. Prior to that time, I had only reluctantly shed a few tears in secret, for I remembered well my mother's remonstrance, "If you cry, I'll give you something to cry about." While in treatment, I watched in wonderment and envy as others were held and nurtured as their tears flowed. But I held back. "You have to be strong," played my childhood tape. Finally, my internal dam broke and, for the first time in my life, I was lovingly held as I cried to the depth of my being.

Have you ever refused to cry because you didn't know why you wanted to cry? In my trauma recovery, I learned to cry into the feeling and, as my tears flowed, I often inwardly viewed a movie reel of one or more incidents that were the source of my pain. By crying into my pain, I received new trauma memories or experienced collective grieving of old wounds.

Following trauma treatment, I was a raw wound. For distance between me and my perpetrators, I left Oklahoma and took a job with the Indian Health Service in Alaska. I needed time to heal and make sense of the pieces of my life.

My first Alaskan winter was my dark night of the soul. The winter was long, cold, dark, and lonely, but it forced me to reach deep into myself and walk close to God. I hurt, cried, prayed, meditated, and worked. During that time, my patients were my salvation. In helping them heal their hurts and wounds, mine healed.

Oftentimes, when we are in pain, we feel we have nothing to give others. Actually, our most important gift to others is sharing who we are, which includes our pain, sorrow, and healing.

After releasing our tears and moving through our pain, we become a beacon of inspiration to others. I met such a person one December morning, when I had to leave my car at the dealership for repairs and take a taxi to work. After settling into the taxi, I was greeted by a portly and loquacious driver, Fred, who related to me his Christmas joy.

Each Christmas Fred dons gear and becomes Santa Claus to many. Fred regaled me with the many events he attended, including the Governor's Christmas Party. Fred shared the joy he received by giving to others and said he refused to take a fee for his services but, if they insisted, he requested they use the money to purchase toys that he might distribute to the needy.

In my usual fashion, I began to ask Fred about his wife and children. He then stated, "You might as well know the rest of the story." Fred related, seven years earlier, his two children, ages two and four, and his wife were killed in an automobile accident. In his grief and anguish, Fred said he spent the next two years in the "nut ward" and was only now able to consider the possibility of remarrying and having children.

Fred went on to say, "If you want a blessing, be one; life is what you give, and the important stuff comes when you are not looking." Through God's healing love, Fred had transformed his grief into a blessing for all he met. As I stepped from the taxi, I felt a skip in my step and knew I had just taken a sleigh ride with Kris Kringle.

Before one can know deep joy, one must often feel deep pain. Relinquish your control. Surrender to your pain and tears and move through your dark night of the soul. It seems only after having lived through the darkness can one truly appreciate the light.

MISERY

Although painful events are a necessary part of life, misery is optional. If we choose recovery, we feel our pain, cry our tears to the marrow of our beings, then move on down life's adventurous road. However, too often, I have seen individuals stay stuck in their pain and relish their victimhood. While hanging on their cross, they continually rehash, to anyone that will listen, their litany of past, present, and anticipated future woes.

I once saw a man so enamored with his life injuries, it was like observing an infant playing in the contents of his dirty diaper. Since it was late on a Friday afternoon and his chart was six inches thick, I stated that I was not interested in all his past life wounds, but I was very interested in what he was doing to change his current life circumstances. Enraged, the fifty-year-old "King Baby" stormed out of the office.

We may have been victims in our childhood. However, if we continue to harm ourselves by our choices, we are no longer victims, but volunteers. I help people through their pain and grief. If they want to wallow in it, I refuse to participate, because I know that pain is a necessary part of life, but misery is totally optional.

INVENTORY

When anger, fear, and pain overwhelm us, it is often necessary to inventory past and present thoughts, feelings, and behaviors and examine how they contributed to creating the contents of our emotional storehouse.

As my patients inventory their lives, I frequently write down their exact words. I know, if I listen carefully, they will give me their answers. In an unguarded moment, they will drop clues in a word or phrase, which unlocks the door to the hidden messages stored in their subconscious mind.

I once worked with a thrice-divorced woman in her twenties. She listed a number of characteristics that attracted her to a man. All but one of these characteristics were indicative of someone who could form mature long-term relationships. However, the outlier was the "pitter patter." On further examination, it became apparent that her primary attraction to a man was the "pitter patter," and this quality occurred only with the excitement of a new relationship.

Along similar lines, I listened as a man in pain repeatedly stated that he had to "suck it up." Actually, the opposite was true. He needed to "let it out." The former phrase reinforced his belief that he had to be strong, not feel, keep control, and know the answers. Conversely, his emotional health lay down the path of let it go, be human, feel, not know the answers, and let God be his strength and solution.

Words are so powerful that they can alter our life's course. For instance, I often hear men who cannot achieve an erection refer to themselves, with lowered heads of resignation, as "impotent." We begin by examining the word impotent, which is defined as, "Lacking power, strength, or vigor: helpless; or unable to copulate." Copulate is defined as, "To engage in sexual intercourse, and intercourse is defined as, "Physical sexual contact between individuals that involves the genitalia of at least one person." By these definitions, a man can "copulate" or have "intercourse" without an erect penis. There are many ways a man can give and receive sexual and emotional pleasure to and from his partner, with or without an erect penis. Therefore, it is reasonable to conclude that a man's power, strength, vigor, and manhood has nothing to do with the firmness of his penis.

As we inventory our thoughts and subsequent emotions and behaviors, we become aware that we have wronged others and owe amends. Have you ever said or done something that you knew was wrong, but your pride would not allow you to admit it? Did you feel a burden from those unspoken amends or untold secrets? As you procrastinated on righting the wrong, did you feel like you were carrying a sack of rocks uphill?

When we carry around unconfessed misdeeds, they develop into heavy loads of shame and guilt. When we finally confess our wrongs and make amends to those we have harmed, we feel lighter, there is a bounce in our step, and our heads are erect.

For our emotional, spiritual, and physical health, we must inventory and cleanse the warehouse of our minds. As we search each shelf and cranny, we discover antiquated or toxic thoughts and beliefs and their resultant feelings. We can give a heave-ho to some of these thoughts and feelings, others may require processing with wise counsel, and others still need to be discussed directly with those personally involved. In the latter, communication skills are necessary for the most constructive outcome of such discussions.

EMOTIONAL COMMUNICATION

In the constructive communication of feelings, I have found the following phrases to be invaluable:

When you_____, I feel_____
_____.

No one can argue with a feeling. This phrasing puts the focus on how one feels about another's words or behaviors and avoids the use of "You did this_____"
statements, which are judgmental or accusatory.

What did you mean when you said_____
_____?
When you said_____, I heard_____
_____.
My perception is_____
_____.

Clarifying communication in this form inventories each other's reality. We can all hear and see the same thing but have entirely different perceptions of their meaning. This form of communication deletes the error of assuming what another is thinking or feeling.

Are you willing to_____?
I am willing to_____.

I am not willing to_____.

Few people appreciate being commanded. With this phrasing, one is asked and given choices. Notice, the word "want" is absent. Often, we may not want to do something, but we are willing to.

Is it possible that_____?
Do you suppose_____?
I wonder _____?

This phrasing invites the exploration of possibilities and choices. It avoids the dogmatic declaration of one person's interpretation as fact.

When all else fails:
We can agree to disagree.

With this statement, no one is right or wrong. No one wins or loses. You just agree to disagree.

Also, in communicating with oneself or others, consider deleting the shaming and condemning words "should" and ought."

In communication, the phrases we use determine whether we are armed for battle or can calmly discuss difficult topics, so put down your weapons and choose your words carefully.

We often live our lives oblivious to our thoughts that result in fearful, angry, and painful feelings and destructive actions. When our lives run amok or become intolerable, we may finally stop and inventory our mental warehouse. Because what we have stored there determines our life.

CHAPTER SIXTEEN

Our Spirits

Our life's purpose is to evolve spiritually and to help others to evolve spiritually. The inward path to our divine Self and its union with God is found through prayer, meditation, and aligning our will with God's. Divine Will is revealed to us in times of quiet contemplation and comes in the form of inner promptings or intuitive knowings.

GOD'S PLAN

My first inkling that God had a plan for me came when I was sixteen and the band's head twirler. It was a Friday night before a home football game. I was severely depressed, felt fat and ugly, and couldn't bear the idea of prancing to music in a short skirt. I went to the bathroom and took a large quantity of pills. I thought of taking more, but decided, no, if what I had taken wouldn't do it, nothing would. I told my mother that I was sick and went to bed. From a deep sleep, my mother roused me and forced me to go to the game. I performed all evening in a drugged stupor.

In the meantime, my mother discovered the pills were missing from the medicine cabinet. When I arrived home, she gave me a tongue lashing then rushed me to the local hospital. As I lay in a semi-conscious state, I heard the doctor tell my parents that it was too late to pump my stomach. He didn't expect me to live. But as I lay there, I wondered why they were so upset, because at that moment I knew, without a doubt, God had a plan for my life, and it was not my time to die.

As God's plan unfolded in my life, I learned that, "Everything is in Divine right order, even if I don't like or understand the order." This principle was often demonstrated to me on my call nights during the Alaskan winters. When the phone rang, I was required to leave my warm bed, get in my cold truck, and make the trek to the hospital emergency room. On those nights, I always prayed for, "Thy will not mine be done," because I sure as heck knew it was not my will to be out on a night like that. But so often, the patient I was called to see was one who touched my heart and, on my way home, I felt that warm glow that comes from knowing that God's plans far outshine my own.

In seeking God's plan, I work to align my will with God's, and my often repeated prayer is, "God, show me the way." When that knowing of God's will comes, I initially may feel resistance, but I have learned to shrug off my schedule and simply say, "Thy will not mine be done," "Such is life," or "Whatever."

These phrases speak to me of acceptance and letting go and surrendering to God's plan. These phrases also speak to me of my lack of control over people, places, things, and situations. When you feel yourself tighten up on life's steering wheel, let go. When you feel yourself trying to direct life's traffic, go sit on a park bench and say, "Whatever...such is life," or "Thy will not mine be done." Then, watch how God resolves the traffic jams.

For my marching orders, God has many ways of getting my attention. For example, I am not much of a mechanic, and sometimes my best solution is to give something a good whack with a hammer. You would be surprised how often that works. Sometimes I think God does the same thing with me. When I get off in life's ditch, God gives me a good whack with life's hammer to set me back on my appointed road.

When I pursue my will, I often feel as though I am being bloodied and beaten by circumstances or my thoughts and feelings toward them. However, if I persist through prayer and meditation to do the next right thing, I later see clearly why I received God's redirection.

So, when you feel as though you have just been whacked by life's hammer, you might consider it is God's way of getting your attention. After you are out of the ditch and back on God's road, you may understand the reason for the painful cue and be grateful for your realignment.

When I followed my plan, I spent much of my time working hard for second best. When I finally began to surrender to God's plan, I realized God wants the best for me, but I must be willing to let go of control. I have struggled many times to make a situation, job, or relationship follow my schedule but, after exhausting myself and finally letting go of control, the issues resolved while I was sleeping. On awakening in my life, I am presented with marvelous solutions underscored with God's signature.

ACCEPTANCE

When I let go of my expectations and accept life on life and God's terms, I am peaceful. When I have high expectations of myself or others, my serenity goes out the window.

We often fret, worry, struggle, push, and pull to get some-one or something to follow our direction. We often expect our spouse, child, home, or ourself to look, do, or be a certain way in our striving to reach unrealistic or unobtainable goals. As we tire ourselves and others in these fruitless efforts, we may notice tension in our neck and shoulders and a knot in our stomach. Stop. Resign from being your life's producer and director.

To reach a state of acceptance when things aren't going ac-cording to your script, consider using the "Serenity Prayer."

"God, grant me the serenity to accept the things I cannot change, the courage to change the things I can, and the wisdom to know the difference."

"God, grant me the serenity" to accept life on life's terms.

"God, grant me...the courage to change the things I can." The only thing we can change is ourselves, our thoughts, and actions, and we need God's help to do that.

"God, grant me...the wisdom to know the difference." Wisdom comes from God as we release, surrender, and listen to our spiritual teachers and inner knowings.

So, when you find yourself troubled, say the "Serenity Prayer," and act with serenity, courage, and wisdom.

Likewise, when our expectations begin to rise, we may ask ourselves, "Compared to my peace of mind, how important is it really?" When we surrender our self-will and accept that God is large and in charge, we can let go of our expectations and accept people, places, and things on life and God's terms.

EGO

On observing a psychiatrist introduce the word "EGO," one might expect a Freudian dissertation. Wrong.

In some spheres, the human ego is described as the false self. This ego self is driven by fear and the ego's attachment to the external world of power, prestige, and possessions. This is contrasted to the inner world of the divine Self and its communion with God.

In twelve-step programs, the "EGO," stands for "Easing God Out." In these programs, members speak of individuals with compulsive-addictive behaviors as "egomaniacs, with inferiority complexes." In contrast, program members speak of "humility" as "being teachable...being right size."

Regarding the latter definition, I found a wonderful metaphor one summer while picking blackberries. I noticed that the most succulent and beautiful berries were found on the lowest, darkest, and most secluded branches. To see and obtain these lovely berries, I had to kneel and look up.

So often, in prideful, egotistical stances, we feel we can see more from lofty perches. This is not the case with the Oklahoma blackberry. Few berries are gathered from pride's lofty perch. But with a humble stance, one receives the most succulent and bountiful fruit.

How many times in your life, in an inflated ego state, have you been unteachable? Did it take one of life's thumps on the head to get your attention? You might consider making things easier for yourself. Be teachable. Be right size. Humble yourself and ease God into your life.

PRAYER

Once on driving through East Texas, I saw a church sign reading, "Don't limit God." I don't know about you, but when I pray, I get better results if I pray, "Thy will, not mine, be done." If I give God a laundry list of requests, directions, and solutions, I shortchange myself.

Before learning to pray for God's will instead of mine, I always settled for crumbs and second best. I now know my God wants only the best for me, but I have to give God free rein and not place limits with my thinking or my praying.

When I place no limit on God in my praying and turn all of my life over to God's care, the obstacles in my life disappear. This is particularly true when my thoughts generate feelings of anger or resentment toward those I think have wronged me. For relief from the discomfort of these feelings, I pray for these individuals to be surrounded by God's light, love, and blessings, whether I mean it or not.

An example of such prayer followed the theft of my two generators. One night while driving home, I realized my life was being polluted by the resentment I felt toward those nameless, faceless individuals. For relief, I knew that I needed to pray for them, and I definitely did not want to. I proceeded to pray for them. However, the prayer began with an expletive on their birth. From much practice, I have found daily prayer, even prayers that begin in this manner, will work.

Goodness knows, I would have appreciated the thieves having a change of heart and miraculously returning my generators and apologizing for my inconvenience. However, the purpose of the prayer is to relieve me of the resentment that, if not removed, would fester in my soul.

So, for many nights afterward, before going to bed, I got on my knees and prayed for those folks and, eventually, I prayed without an exclamation on their birth. Soon thereafter, my anger and resentment had peacefully vanished. On some level, I accepted that those individuals needed the generators more than I did.

As we pray, our prayers are answered in many ways. My friend, David, once recounted to me his experience with prayer and a radio.

David said that he was going through a dark time in his life. One night, he was driving his semitrailer truck between Washington, D.C., and Baltimore, and he prayed for God to show him a "sign." He wanted to know "if there was some light at the end of this long, dark tunnel?" He had a radio that had not worked for years. On the return trip, the radio light came on, and the radio began to play.

Have you ever experienced a dark night of the soul and sent out a prayer for a sign, and the sign came? We often go along in a bleak and lonely existence and do not call on God's love for solace, when all that is needed is a simple prayer, like David's on his lonely night between Washington, D.C. and Baltimore. The night the radio came on.

An excellent guideline for prayer is the eleventh step in twelve-step programs which reads, "Sought through prayer and meditation to improve our conscious contact with God, praying only for the knowledge of His will for us and the power to carry it out."

How wonderfully simple. One prays "only for the knowledge of His will.. .and the power to carry it out." For me, there
is an implicit promise in this kind of prayer. When I receive the
knowledge of God's will and choose to follow God's direction, I
will be given the power to carry it out. You can't beat a deal like
that.

Prayer has been described as "talking to God" and meditation as "listening to God." In times of deep pain and confusion, I
go to God in prayer. I then wait and listen as God reveals where
to place my feet one step at a time. God does not disclose my
destination, because I might balk or attempt to take control. As
the steps unfold, it is like the parting of the Red Sea.

So when you are at your Red Sea, and the enemy is at your
back, pray for the knowledge of God's will, listen, and watch the
waters part.

MEDITATION

In listening for God in meditation, some would have us believe that one meditates only when one is on their knees or in a
lotus position, chanting or floating off into sublime quiet.

I have moments of the purest, sweetest insight while meditat-
ing on the bathroom throne, gardening, mowing grass, walking,
washing dishes, or taking a shower. During these moments, the
mind's chatter diminishes, and the pure sweetness of our inner
truth and its divine connection is revealed. I have wisely been
told, "The sacred is in the ordinary." Therefore, it is possible that
one's enlightenment can be found there.

Certainly, I am aware there are many advanced forms of meditation handed down to us by enlightened masters. However,

the ordinary tasks of life are sacred and are a form of meditation. Other forms of meditation include reading sacred writings and listening to elevating music. Meditation includes any method that silences the outer world, quiets the mind, and allows us to go inward and access the Divine.

In meditation, our answers to life's dilemmas are revealed. Unfortunately, we are a nation of intellectuals and left-brainers that believe if we or others think hard enough and long enough, our brains will figure out the answers to most of life's problems.

Contrary to that opinion, the answers often come when we stop thinking and begin listening to our inner knowing or intuition that is felt in our hearts or our guts. You will often hear others speak of their inner knowing in terms of, "In my heart, I don't know how, but I know it's true," or "In the pit of my stomach, it just feels right." Often we are so busy looking for the answers in our cerebral cortex or someone else's that we overlook our most valuable source of information—our intuition.

With meditation and prayer, we quiet our brain's chatter and inwardly listen for the Divine Voice. So, when you find yourself frenziedly scurrying, looking for answers in books, on the Internet, or in other people's brains, stop, be quiet, look within, trust your gut, and listen to your heart.

Like many others, I was reared in an atmosphere of constant criticism and was frequently demeaned if I didn't know the answer to a question or how to do something. Naturally, I grew up thinking it was my job to know the answers. Of course, being human, I was doomed to failure. What a relief to learn to rely on God and find it was not my job to know all the answers, especially when I didn't even know the questions. I have learned my job is to align my will with God's, put my life in God's care, and listen for God's answers through prayer and meditation.

GOD'S HUMOR

In all the gravity and seriousness of life, I have come to realize that my God has a wonderful sense of humor. For instance, on the night that God's messenger came to me in the form of an RV park manager, I had prayed for a new home for my dog, Sam, because I knew he was causing difficulty in the trailer park. After the irate manager beat on my door at 2:00 a.m., I was hitching the trailer to the truck and began to laugh. I realized that before going to bed the preceding evening, I had prayed for a new home for Sam, little knowing I was going to get one too.

God's humor was also evident after the theft of my generators. While discussing my theft with neighbors, I said in jest that I needed "a half-dozen rottweilers." On a stormy night two weeks later, there came to the farm Mama and her eight puppies, five with rottweiler marking.

As do my rural neighbors, my God seems to have a country-like, belly-laughing sense of the absurd, and I am frequently delighted by God's humor.

GOD'S WISDOM

God's wisdom is infinite. After witnessing many of God's solutions, I determined that I think in straight lines, and God thinks in circles and curves. I finally realized I cannot understand an infinite God with my finite mind.

In my finite thinking, I believe to get from point A to point B is a straight line. Sometimes I presume to use my linear thinking to determine who will recover but, deep down, I know that domain is between God and the individual. When I work with addicts and alcoholics, I think if they go to alcohol and drug treatment they have a good chance of staying sober and clean. However, it often doesn't work that way. God's route is much more circuitous.

This fact was demonstrated to me one morning when I was called by the parents of a twenty-year-old whom I had seen two weeks previously. After our appointment, the young man had returned to his home in Louisiana and stayed drunk for several days. In a blackout, he placed his head on a railroad track. By one of God's miracles, after one-hundred-and-fifty stitches in his head and several fractured neck vertebrae, he was alive, talking coherently, and moving all limbs. Now you figure it.

The young man had already been to several alcohol treatment centers. However, after his suicide attempt and many more months in treatment, he was again drinking and headed home to Oklahoma. On a Saturday night, after crossing the border into Texas, his tire blew. Without a spare, he had to wait until the next morning for his tire repair. He was in a dry county. Something happened. Sober, he came home.

In sobriety, the young man put himself through college with honors, married, and now has a young son. Only God could have known this young man's sobriety would come from a flat tire on a Saturday night in a dry county in Texas.

I cannot understand an infinite God with my finite mind. I think in straight lines, but my God thinks in circles and curves.

In God's infinite wisdom, God works on God's time schedule. Some ask, "How fast does God work?" Others reply, "Right behind Methuselah." Have you ever prayed and prayed for an answer to a problem, and the answer would not come, or the answer was "wait?" Have you ever worked long and hard toward a goal, but the goal eluded you? It often seems God is giving us a wake-up call about who is in charge of the scheduling department, and it's not us.

Sometimes, when I am demanding an answer, I set up the dominoes in the way I think they should fall. When the long awaited solution comes, I see that all along, God had been aligning the cosmic dominoes to fall in a way I could never have conceived.

God's wisdom is present in every aspect of our lives. For example on my farm, I have a lot of brush and trees, and I enjoy clearing the underbrush and pruning the trees of their dead and excess branches. Pruning reveals the tree's character and beauty. With infinite wisdom, God prunes us the same way. We often hold onto dead or excess parts of ourselves or our lives, but these must be shed to allow our divine Self to emerge.

In our pruning, we must trust God's wisdom and become "entirely ready" and "humbly ask" God to remove these dead or excess parts of ourselves. So, when you hold tightly to behaviors, thoughts, or situations and find yourself becoming uncomfortable, release yourself to the infinite wisdom of the Master Pruner.

Sometimes in our pruning, our emotional pain is so great that we feel like our hide is being ripped off. I believe to the depth of my being, "Nothing, absolutely nothing, happens in God's world by mistake," and that includes emotional pain. That hide-ripping kind of pain requires us to go to the depth of our being, surrender, and grow. I don't need to understand God's plan, but usually in retrospect, I see from that pain flourished new growth.

Have you ever seen pink, healthy, fresh, new skin growing after the superficial layers were removed? This is exactly the process found in the high-dollar world of plastic surgery, with peels, scrapes, and lasers. So, when you are emotionally hurting and feel as if your hide has been ripped off, remember, in God's infinite wisdom you are just getting a little surgery of the soul, without the plastic.

There were times in my spiritual journey that I was in such emotional pain that I knew I had to make a change or die. I felt like I was backed to the edge of a cliff on a black, stormy night, and the only way I could save my life was to jump, so I did. Each time, God caught me and placed me on a rich new path, the likes of which I could not have even imagined. To avoid change, I was often dragged kicking and screaming to these defining moments. Over and over, I jumped and, each time I did, my life got better. Slowly, I developed a deep faith in God's infinite love and wisdom.

So, when you are backed up to your emotional cliff, jump. Only then can you develop faith that God will catch you in the most creative of ways.

I absolutely trust God's infinite wisdom. No matter what befalls me or others, I believe something good will come of it. My God is all-knowing, all-powerful, all-loving, and wants only the best for all concerned. I cannot comprehend God's plan with my finite mind but, if I look, even in the most seemingly horrible of circumstances, I can find some good and that gives me peace.

I believe in God's love even in the death of a child. Who am I to know in the birth of a child what is that child's destiny? Who am I to know what is important for that child to do in their lifetime?

I once heard a man in his forties discuss the birth of his only child, twenty years earlier. The child lived two days, but the bond and love between the man and his son indelibly touched his life. For that brief moment, the man knew absolute unconditional love. Perhaps touching this man was that child's sole mission in life? I do not know, but that thought gives me comfort.

DIVINE LOVE

God's infinite love is in every person, place, thing, and situation. We must only look with eyes that see and listen with ears that hear. Several years ago, I found an expression of God's love in Glide Memorial Church, located near the Haight-Asbury region in San Francisco. The church was large, old, and rocked with people and sounds on Sunday morning.

The pastor said, "Everybody is welcome at Glide," and so they were. Glide's doors were open and received everyone from the homeless addict to San Francisco's upper-crust.

The Glide choir swayed to such songs as "God is Good to Me" and "Breaking Free." At Glide, people clapped their hands and danced in the aisles, and under it all was a tone of people breaking free from whatever bound them and, no matter what their bondage, they received love and acceptance at Glide.

With "God is Love," the Glide choir rhythmically belted out:

God is love...He likes to see you with your head held high, even though tears may fall from your eyes...
We have to live our lives the very best we can...
God is love, He's love, He's love...God is love.

So, when your head is bent and the tears are falling, remember, "He likes to see you with your head held high...God is love, He's love, He's love...God is love," and if you are of love, you are of God.

The Glide choir also crooned:

> Today is the first day of the rest of my life...
> I'm going to take it one day at a time...
> first day, first day of my life.

Today, we can start our lives over. We can choose to be the person and live the life God intended. It is our choice. What we choose to think and how we choose to act will determine how we feel and who we become. It is our choice.

Life and the universe are our teachers. Today is the first day of the rest of your life. God invites you to embark on your grand adventure and discover your true Self.

NOTES

1. Yogananda, 1990, 1-6.
2. Mitchell, 8..
3. Taylor, 54, 97.
4. Strehlow, 2002, 59
5. Hawkins, 2001, 317.
6. Roth, 1997, 223.
7. Bowlby, 2006, publication pending.
8. Sellers, 47.
9. Jampolsky, 1970, 18-24, 131.

SUGGESTED READINGS

Alcoholics Anonymous. Alcoholics Anonymous World Services, Inc., New York, New York, 1976.

Beattie, M. *Codependent No More.* Hazelden, Center City, Minnesota, 1987.

Beattie, M. *Codependents' Guide to the Twelve-Steps.* Prentice Hall Press, New York, New York, 1990.

Bee, B. *The Cob Builders Handbook.* Groundworks, Murphy, Oregon, 1997.

Bodenhamer, G. *Parent In Control.* Simon & Schuster, New York, New York, 1995.

Bolen, J. *Crones Don't Whine.* Conari Press, Boston, Massachusetts, 2003.

Borysenko, J. *Fire in the Soul.* Warner Books, New York, New York, 1993.

Bowlby, L. *Red Earth Woman.* Red Earth Inc., Oklahoma City, Oklahoma, 2006.

Bowlby, L. *Renaissance Woman.* Red Earth Inc., Oklahoma City, Oklahoma, 2006.

Browne, J. "You Ain't Down-Home." "Country's Greatest Hits." Volume 4.

Campbell, J. *The Power of Myth.* Anchor Books, New York, New York, 1988.

Carnes, P. *Out of the Shadows.* Compcare Publications, Minneapolis, Minnesota, 1983.

Chernin, K. *The Obsession, Reflections on the Tyranny of Slenderness.* First Harper Colophon, New York, New York, 1981.

Chopra, D. *The Book of Secrets.* Three Rivers Press, New York, New York, 2004.

Cousins, N. *Anatomy of an Illness.* Bantam Books, New York, New York, 1979.

Dyer, W. *The Power of Intention.* Hay House, Carlsband, California, 2004.

Ellis, P. *Border Healing Woman.* Texas University Press, Austin, Texas, 1994.

Emoto, M. *The Hidden Messages in Water.* Beyond Words Publishing, Hillsboro, Oregon, 2004.

Glide Ensemble Tapes. Glide Memorial Church, San Francisco, California.

Gray, J. *Men Are From Mars, Women Are From Venus.* HarperCollins Publishers, New York, New York, 1992.

Hawkins, D. *Power Vs. Force.* HayHouse, Inc., Carlsbad, California, 2002.

Hawkins, D. *The Eye of the I.* Veritas, West Sedona, Arizona, 2001.

Hawkins, D. *I.* Veritas, West Sedona, Arizona, 2003.

Hay, L. *The Power Is Within You.* Hay House, Carson, California, 1991.

Hay, L. *You Can Heal Your Life.* Hay House, Santa Monica, California, 1984.

Jampolsky, G. *Teach Only Love.* Bantam Books, New York, New York, 1970.

Jampolsky, G. *Love Is Letting Go of Fear.* Bantam Books, New York, New York, 1979.

Lipton, B. *The Biology of Belief.* Spirit 2000, Inc., Video Series distributed by Spirit 2000, Inc.

Lipton, B. *The Biology of Belief.* Mountain of Love/ Elite Books, Santa Rosa, California, 2005.

Martin, H. *The Secret Teachings of the Espiritistas.* Metamind Publicatons, Savannah, Georgia, 1998.

Mitchell, S. *Tao Te Ching, A New English Version.* Harper Collins Publishers, Inc., New York, New York, 1992.

Nerburn, K. *Make Me an Instrument of Your Peace.* HarperCollins Publishers, New York, New York, 1999.

Norwood, R. *Women Who Love too Much.* Pocket Books, New York, New York, 1985.

Reynolds, M. *Earthship, Volume 1.* Solar Survival Press, Taos, New Mexico, 1993.

Roth, G. *Breaking Free From Compulsive Eating.* Penguin Press, New York, New York, 1984.

Roth, G. *When You Eat at the Refrigerator, Pull Up a Chair.* Hyperion, New York, New York, 1998.

Roth, R. *The Healing Path of Prayer.* Three Rivers Press, New York, New York, 1997.

Roth, R. *Prayer and the Five Stages of Growth.* Hay House, Carlsbad, California, 1999.

Roth, R. *Holy Spirit; The Boundless Energy of God.* Hay House, Carlsbad, California, 2000.

Roth, R. *Reclaim Your Spiritual Power.* Hay House, Carlsbad, California, 2002.

Sellers, B. *Unique Effects of Alcoholism in Women.* Primary Psychiatry, January, 2005, 47-50.

Siegel, B. *Love, Medicine, and Miracles.* Harper and Row Publishers, New York, New York, 1986.

Siegel, B. *Peace, Love, and Healing.* Walker Publishing Company, New York, New York, 1990.

Siegel, B. *Prescriptions for Living.* Quill, New York, New York, 1998.

Siegel, B. *Help Me to Heal.* Hay House, Carlsbad, California, 2003.

Siegel, B. *365 Prescriptions for the Soul.* New World Library, Novato, California, 2004.

Steen, A. *Straw Bale House.* Chelsea Publishing Company, White River Junction, Vermont, 1994.

Strehlow, W. *Hildegard of Bingen's Spiritual Remedies.* Healing Arts Press, Rochester, Vermont, 2002.

Taylor, P. *Border Healing Woman.* University of Texas Press, Austin, Texas, 1981.

Tolle, E. *A New Earth.* Dutton, New York, New York, 2005.

Twelve Steps and Twelve Traditions. Alcoholics Anonymous World Service, Inc., New York, New York, 1981.

Uhlein, G. *Meditations With Hildegard of Bingen.* Bear and Company Publishing, Santa Fe, New Mexico, 1983.

Webster, M. *Webster's New Collegiate Dictionary.* G.&C. Merriam Company, Springfield, Massachusetts, 1980.

Wegscheider-Cruse, S. *Choice-Making.* Health Communications, Inc., Pompano Beach, Florida, 1985.

Whitfield, C. *Healing the Child Within.* Health Communications, Inc., Pompano Beach, Florida, 1987.

Wilson-Schaef, A. *Codependence, Misunderstood-Mistreated.* Winston Press, Minneapolis, Minnesota, 1986.

Woititz, J. *Adult Children of Alcoholics.* Health Communications, Inc., Pompano Beach, Florida, 1983.

Woititz, J. *Struggle for Intimacy.* Health Communications, Inc., Pompano Beach, Florida, 1986.

Yogananda, P. *Where There is Light.* Self-Realization Fellowship, Los Angeles, California, 1988.

Yogananda, P. *The Essence of Self-Realization.* Crystal Clarity Publishers, Nevada City, California, 1990.

Yogananda, P. *In the Sanctuary of the Soul.* Self-Realization Fellowship, Los Angeles, California, 1998.